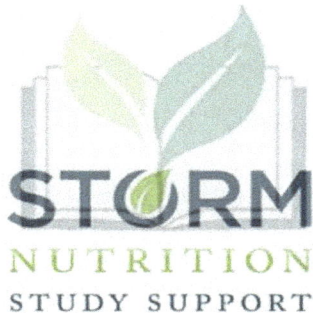

STORM
NUTRITION
STUDY SUPPORT

PARENTERAL NUTRITION

TRAINING GUIDE

2nd Edition

STORM NUTRITION STUDY SUPPORT

Bridget Storm, MA, RD-AP, LDN, CNSC

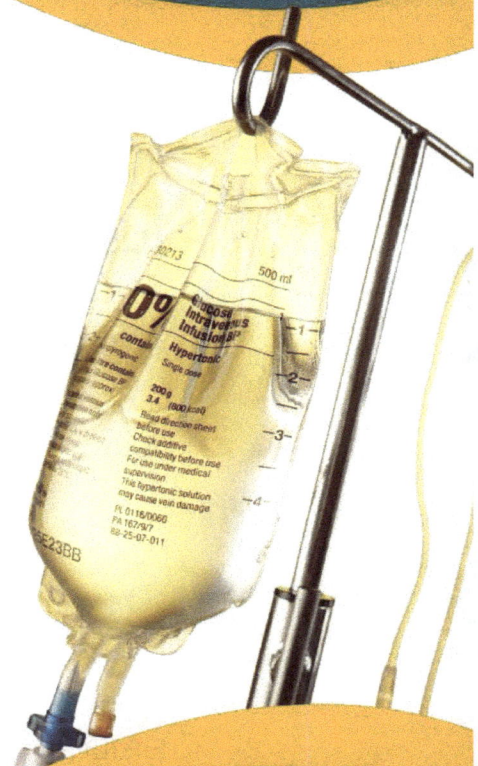

https://nutritionstudysupport.com

"You Don't Have to See the Whole Staircase, Just to Take the First Step."

-    *Martin Luther King, Jr.*

PARENTERAL NUTRITION TRAINING GUIDE

BRIDGET STORM, MA, RD-AP, LDN, CNSC
STORM NUTRITION STUDY SUPPORT
Copyright © 2024 *(Updated 2026)*
ISBN# 979-8-9903170-7-9 *eBook/pdf*; ISBN# 979-8-9903170-6-2 *print*

Contents:

FLUID & ELECTROLYTE MANAGEMENT

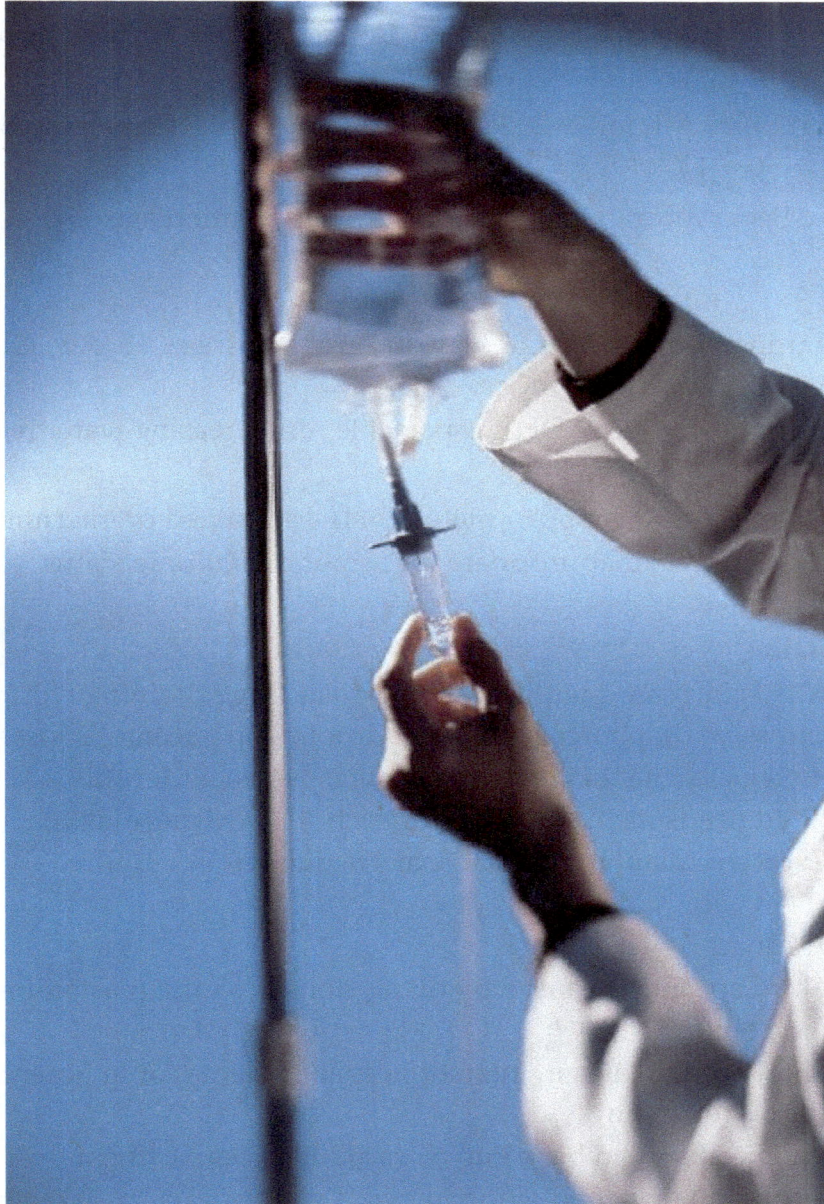

FLUID & ELECTROLYTE MANAGEMENT

FLUID REQUIREMENTS

Age < 50 years	1500 ML for 1st 20 kg Body Wt + [20 ML × Remaining Body Wt (kg)]
Age > 50 years	1500 ML for 1st 20 kg Body Wt + [15 ML × Remaining Body Wt (kg)]

- Holliday-Segar recommended to prevent dehydration age 65+

Fluid Balance

- Normal urinary losses 0.8-1.5L/day, insensible losses ~ 1L/day, GI losses 100-200 g stool/day
- Antidiuretic Hormone (ADH) responsible for increasing water reabsorption by kidneys
- SIADH (Symptom of Inappropriate ADH) – sustained or intermittently elevated ADH level inappropriate for osmotic & volume status

- Dehydration
  - Needs increased with severe diarrhea, large draining wounds, excessive diaphoresis, constant drooling, paracentesis losses, drains, high gastric/fistula/ostomy outputs, persistent fevers
  - Fluid needs increase by 7% for each °F above normal
  - Excessive diaphoresis that soaks bed linens is ~ 1L fluid

- Fluid Overload
  - Third spacing is caused by disruptions favoring plasma-to- interstitial fluid shift
  - Fluid accumulates in interstitial space (edema) or in potential fluid spaces (effusion)
  - Will be absorbed back into extracellular compartment over days to weeks but acute reduction in blood volume can cause severe dehydration
  - Common in critical illness due to increased capillary permeability

IV (INTRAVENOUS) FLUIDS

- Lactated Ringers (LR), Normal Saline (NS) & Normosol-R are isotonic & can be used for resuscitation
- Normal Saline (NS) is 0.9% NaCl
- Isotonic NS is 3x more efficient than D5W at expanding extracellular space
- D5 & ½ NS are hypotonic and used for hypernatremia/increased free water need
- 3% NaCl is hypertonic and used by Neurology in brain injury

Electrolyte Content of IV Solutions								
	Na mEq/L	Cl mEq/L	K mEq/L	Ca mEq/L	Mg mEq/L	Lactate mEq/L	Dextrose g/L	mOsm/L
D5W	0	0	0	0	0	0	50	252
½ NS 0.45% NaCl	77	77	0	0	0	0	0	154
D5-1/2 NS 0.45% NaCl	77	77	0	0	0	0	50	406
NS 0.9% NaCl	154	154	0	0	0	0	0	308
D5-NS 0.9% NaCl	154	154	0	0	0	0	50	560
LR	130	109	4	3	2	28	0	273
D5-LR	130	109	4	3	2	28	50	525
Normosol R- pH 7.4	140	98	5	0	3	0 lactate (27 acetate)	0	295

FLUID & ELECTROLYTE DISORDERS

- Abnormalities in renal excretion and excessive losses from the GI tract are often primary contributors to electrolyte imbalances
- Secretions from duodenum, ileum, pancreas & bile have greatest Na content
- In chronic electrolyte disorders, patient often asymptomatic & can be harmed by too rapid correction
- Replete Mg before K+ to optimize repletion – K+ rarely corrected if Mg not corrected first

ELECTROLYTE MANAGEMENT

Overview of Roles

- Sodium
  - Principle cation in ECF
  - Regulates ECF volume & water distribution in body
  - Active transport of molecules across cell membranes

- Potassium
  - Major intracellular cation
  - Critical role in cell metabolism, including protein & glycogen synthesis
  - Maintains resting membrane potential & normal neural & muscular function

- Phosphorus
  - Main intracellular ion
  - Roles in bone & cell membrane composition
  - Normal pH maintenance
  - ATP/energy utilization
  - Neurologic function
  - Muscular function (especially myocardium & diaphragm)

- Magnesium
  - Mostly in ICF, 50-60% in bone
  - Essential in enzyme activation
  - Required for maintenance of Na^+-K^+-ATPase pump
  - Neuromuscular transmission
  - Muscle contraction, including cardiac muscle
  - PTH secretion

- Calcium
    - 99% in bones & teeth, <1% in serum
    - Preserves cell membrane integrity
    - Neuromuscular activity
    - Regulates endocrine hormone secretion
    - Hypercalcemia can be an indicator of malignancy

Normal Serum Electrolyte Concentrations

Element	Serum Reference Range
Sodium (Na)	136 – 144 mg/dL
Potassium (K⁺)	3.6 – 5.1 mmol/L
Phosphorus (Phos)	2.4 – 4.7 mg/dL
Magnesium (Mg)	1.8 – 2.5 mg/dL
Calcium (Ca⁺⁺)	8.9 – 10.3 mg/dL

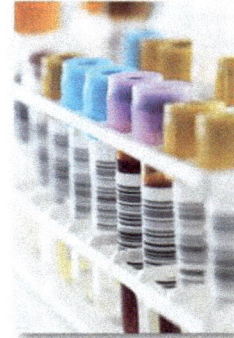

Sodium (Na)

- Principle cation in ECF
- Regulates ECF volume & water distribution in body
- Active transport of molecules across cell membranes

Hyponatremia
- Defined as Na < 135
    - Clinically significant < 130
    - Potential CNS dysfunction < 125
    - ↑ mortality < 120
- Targeted rate of correction to prevent osmotic demyelination:
    - Acute – do not exceed 10-12 mEq/L/d
    - Chronic/unknown duration – do not exceed 6-8 mEq/L/d

Hypotonic Hyponatremia	Characteristics	Causes	Additional Labs	Treatment
Hypovolemic Hypotonic	Lose more sodium in relation to water, fluid retention, concentrated urine	Renal losses/ diuretics, diarrhea, GI fistula output, excessive sweating, burns, open wounds, drains, SAH/ cerebral salt wasting	Urine Osm > Serum Osm Urine Na < 20 mEq/L	Isotonic fluids to expand ECF volume
Euvolemic Hypotonic	Stable Na I/O but retain water d/t excess ADH	SIADH – usually d/t brain/CNS malignancy, head trauma, lung malignancy, PNA Can also be d/t psychogenic polydipsia or hypothyroid	Urine Osm > Serum Osm Urine Na > 20 mEq/L	FR 500-1000 mL Salt tabs Loop diuretics Vasopressin-2 receptor antagonists
Hypervolemic Hypotonic	Fluid retention/3rd spacing, retain more water than Na	End-organ damage (HF, ESRD, ESLD/ ascites)	n/a	Fluid & Na restrictions

Hypernatremia

- Na > 145, significantly ↑ mortality > 160

$$\text{Free Water Deficit} = 0.5 \times IBW \times [1 - (140/\text{Serum Na+})]$$

  - May underestimate FW losses by 1-2.5L, so correlate with clinical signs & symptoms
- Targeted rate of correction to prevent cerebral edema & neurological impairment
  - Acute –2 mEq/L/hr until reach serum Na 145 mEq/L
  - Chronic/unknown duration – do not exceed 10 mEq/L/d

Potassium (K+)

- Major intracellular cation; critical role in cell metabolism, including protein & glycogen synthesis; maintains resting membrane potential & normal neural & muscular function
- Normal daily requirements: 0.5 – 2 mEq/kg

Hypokalemia

- Oral correction safer, less risk of overcorrection or rebound hyperkalemia
- Need 10 mEq K+ for every 0.1 serum increase needed
- IV correction for severe hypokalemia or GI contraindication to po
  - Infusion rates should not exceed 10-20 mEq/hr
  - Total daily supplement should not exceed 40-100 mEq – additional supplementation needs require cardiac monitoring
  - Avoid using dextrose solutions for diluent – can worsen hypokalemia by stimulating insulin release that promotes intracellular K^+ shift
- Mg deficit should be corrected 1st because hypomagnesemia can result in refractory hypokalemia due to accelerated renal K^+ losses or impairment of Na^+-K^+-ATPase pump activity
- Medications can contribute to hypokalemia
  - Albuterol causes potassium to shift into cells
  - Loop diuretics (Lasix, Bumex) are potassium-excreting

Hyperkalemia

- Even small excess of total body K^+ can cause sharp increase in serum levels, but often asymptomatic until > 5.5
- Clinical manifestations cause changes in neuromuscular & cardiac function
- Most often occurs in CKD; also, can be due to certain meds, rhabdomyolysis, metabolic acidosis
- Increased intake alone rarely causes hyperkalemia
- Metabolic acidosis – for every 0.1 ↓ in Ph, K^+ ↑ by average of 0.6 mEq/L (range 0.3-1.3)
- Continue to monitor K+ levels Q4-12 hours after treatment & symptom resolution until levels WNL

- Treatment:
  - Regular insulin & albuterol can treat in 60 minutes
  - Kayexalate & Lokelma take longer (60 minutes) to correct & not acute treatment
  - Calcium gluconate – given concurrently for cardioprotection
  - Severe cases require emergent HD

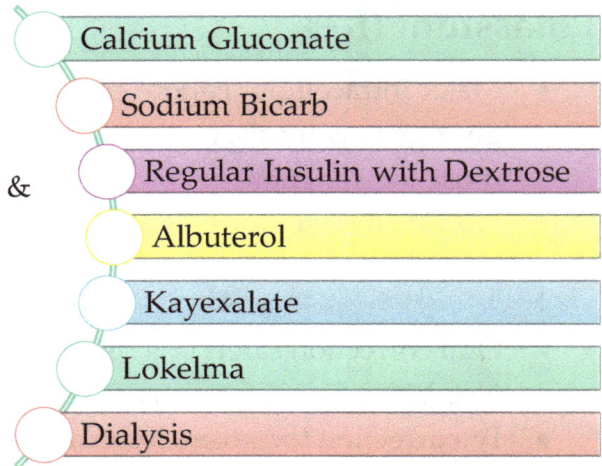

> Calcium Gluconate
> Sodium Bicarb
> Regular Insulin with Dextrose
> Albuterol
> Kayexalate
> Lokelma
> Dialysis

Magnesium (Mg)

- Repletion: IV preferred, infusion rates not to exceed 1 g/hr (8 MEq/hr)
  - Each 1g (8 mEq) should ↑ serum Mg by 0.1 mg/Dl – equilibrium takes up to 48 hours

Calcium (Ca^{2+})

- 99% in bones & teeth, <1% in serum
- Ionized Ca^{2+} is the most accurate assessment of abnormalities because it is not affected by albumin

$$\text{Corrected Total Serum } Ca^{2+} = \text{Measured Total Serum } Ca^{2+} + [0.8 \times (4 - \text{Serum Albumin})]$$

- Repletion
  - $Ca^{2+}Cl$ contains 3x more elemental Ca^{2+} but may cause tissue necrosis if extravasation
  - Ca^{2+} Gluconate recommended repletion (replete Mg first if also low)
  - If due to ↑ Phos, treat with Phos binders first to ↓ risk of soft tissue calcification

Phosphorus (Phos)

- Main intracellular ion, roles in bone & cell membrane composition, normal pH maintenance, ATP/energy utilization, neurologic function, muscular function (especially myocardium & diaphragm)
- Hypophosphatemia
  - Common in alcoholism, critical illness, respiratory & metabolic alkalosis, and following DKA treatment
  - Administration of CHO loads or PN cause hypophosphatemia if inadequate provision or malnourished & at risk of refeeding syndrome
  - Infusion rate should not exceed 7 mmol/hr

> 1 mmol IV K$^+$Phos = 1.47 mEq K$^+$
>
> 1 mmol IV Na Phos = 1.33 mEq Na

Electrolyte Repletion Guide

	Potassium		Magnesium		Phosphorus		Calcium gluconate	
	Serum K$^+$	Repletion	Serum Mg	Repletion	Serum Phos	Repletion	Ionized Ca^{2+}	Repletion
Mild	3.0-3.4	20-40 mEq	1.0-1.5	16-32 mEq (2-4g) Mg sulfate	2.3-2.7	0.08-0.16 mmol/kg	1.0-1.12	1-2g over 1-2 hrs
Moderate	2.5-2.9	40-80 mEq			1.5-2.3	0.16-0.32 mmol/kg		
Severe	<2.5	80-120 mEq	<1.0	32-80 mEq (4-10g) Mg sulfate	<1.5	0.32-1.0 mmol/kg	<1.0	2-4g over 2-4 hrs

Acid-Base Balance

- Normal arterial blood pH = 7.35-7.45
- ABG (arterial blood gas) reflects ability of lungs to oxygenate blood
- VBG (venous blood gas) reflects tissue oxygenation
- HCO_3 = bicarb

Normal Blood Gas Values

	ABG	VBG
pH	7.4 (7.35-7.45)	7.36 (7.31-7.41)
pCO_2	35-45	41-51
pO_2	80-100	35-40
HCO_3-	22-26	24-26

- Metabolic Acidosis uses anion gap to help identify differential diagnosis
  - Normal gap = 9 mEq/L (range 3-11)
  - Low Albumin can falsely decrease AG – for every 1.0 ↓ in Alb, ↓ 2.5-3.0 mEq AG
    - Corrected AG = AG + 2.5 x (4.5 – measured Alb)

- Metabolic Alkalosis – most are saline-responsive (urine Cl^- < 20 mEq/L)
- Chloride: Acetate Ratio in PN start with 1:1 – 1.5:1 in normal balance
  - Risk of metabolic acidosis (AKI, CKD, SB GI bicarb losses) – 1:2 or lower
  - Risk of metabolic alkalosis (gastric losses, volume contraction) – 2:1 or higher
  - Replace base deficit with acetate in PN; generally, add 10mEq acetate per 1 mm/l CO_2 < 24

Compensation

  - Compensation for metabolic disorders starts in minutes
  - Compensation for respiratory disorders fully activated in 2-3 days, often causing delayed AKI
  - Failure to compensate = mixed acid-base disorder → pCO_2 & HCO_3 move in opposite directions

Step-by-step evaluation process

1. Is pH acidic (pH < 7.4) or alkalotic (pH > 7.4)?
   a. If pH is 7.4, mixed acid-base disorder cannot be excluded

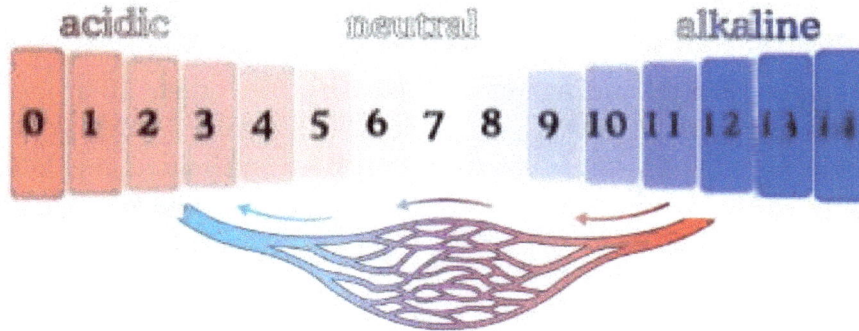

2. Assess PCO_2 for a contributing respiratory process
   a. High PCO_2 → respiratory acidosis
   b. Low PCO_2 → respiratory alkalosis
3. Assess HCO_3^- for contributing metabolic process
   a. High HCO_3^- → metabolic alkalosis
   b. Low HCO_3^- → metabolic acidosis
4. Calculate the anion gap to confirm metabolic acidosis

$$\text{Anion Gap (AG)} = [\text{Serum Na}^+] - ([\text{Serum Cl}^-] + [\text{Serum HCO}_3^-])$$

5. Determine if acute or chronic and if appropriately compensated
6. If compensation is not appropriate, the patient has mixed acid-base disorder

Summary:

Respiratory problem	→ Kidneys fix it
Metabolic/kidney problem	Respiratory System fixes it
↑ Upper GI output	→ Lose Acid
↑ Lower GI output	Lose Base

Condition	Pathophysiology	Lab Values	Compensatory Changes	Treatment
METABOLIC ACIDOSIS	↑ bicarb losses GI losses Kidney/AKI/ATN Lactic acidosis Starvation/drugs ↑ ketones/DKA	↓pH ↓ pCO_2 ↓HCO_3 (all down) ↑K^+ (out of cell)	RESPIRATORY ALKALOSIS ↑ ventilation to ↑ pH Hyperventilation causes ↑ CO_2 elimination Kidneys conserve bicarb	Treat underlying condition Keep K^+ WNL ↓ Cl in TPN ↑acetate (if bicarb losses) Correct acidosis to prevent PRO catabolism & bone loss
METABOLIC ALKALOSIS	↑ H^+ loss from ECF (NG) Use of bicarb precursors (LR, antacids) ↑ loss of Cl (diuretics) Severe K^+ depletion Cushing's disease, hyperaldosteronism	↑pH ↑ pCO_2 ↑HCO_3 (all up) ↓K^+ (shift into cell)	RESPIRATORY ACIDOSIS Hypoventilation causes ↓ pCO_2 & ↑ pH Kidneys ↑ bicarb excretion	D/C diuretics Replace Cl losses Avoid HCO_3 & precursors Use H2 blockers to ↓ gastric acid secretion
RESPIRATORY ACIDOSIS	Hypoventilation CO_2 retention Respiratory distress (CNS depressions, lung disease, COPD, PNA, PE, OSA, stroke, head injury, cardiac arrest, overdose, neuromuscular disease)	↓pH ↑ pCO_2 ↑HCO_3 ↑K^+	METABOLIC ALKALOSIS ↑ reabsorption of HCO_3 to ↑ pH	Avoid overfeeding of total kcal
RESPIRATORY ALKALOSIS	Hyperventilation ↑ elimination of CO_2 Head trauma, brain tumor, PNA, PE, sepsis, fever, HE, cirrhosis, drug use, anxiety, 3rd trimester pregnancy	↑pH ↓ pCO_2 ↓HCO_3	METABOLIC ACIDOSIS ↑ excretion of HCO_3 to ↓ pH	Treat underlying condition Avoid HCO_3 & precursors

PARENTERAL NUTRITION SUPPORT

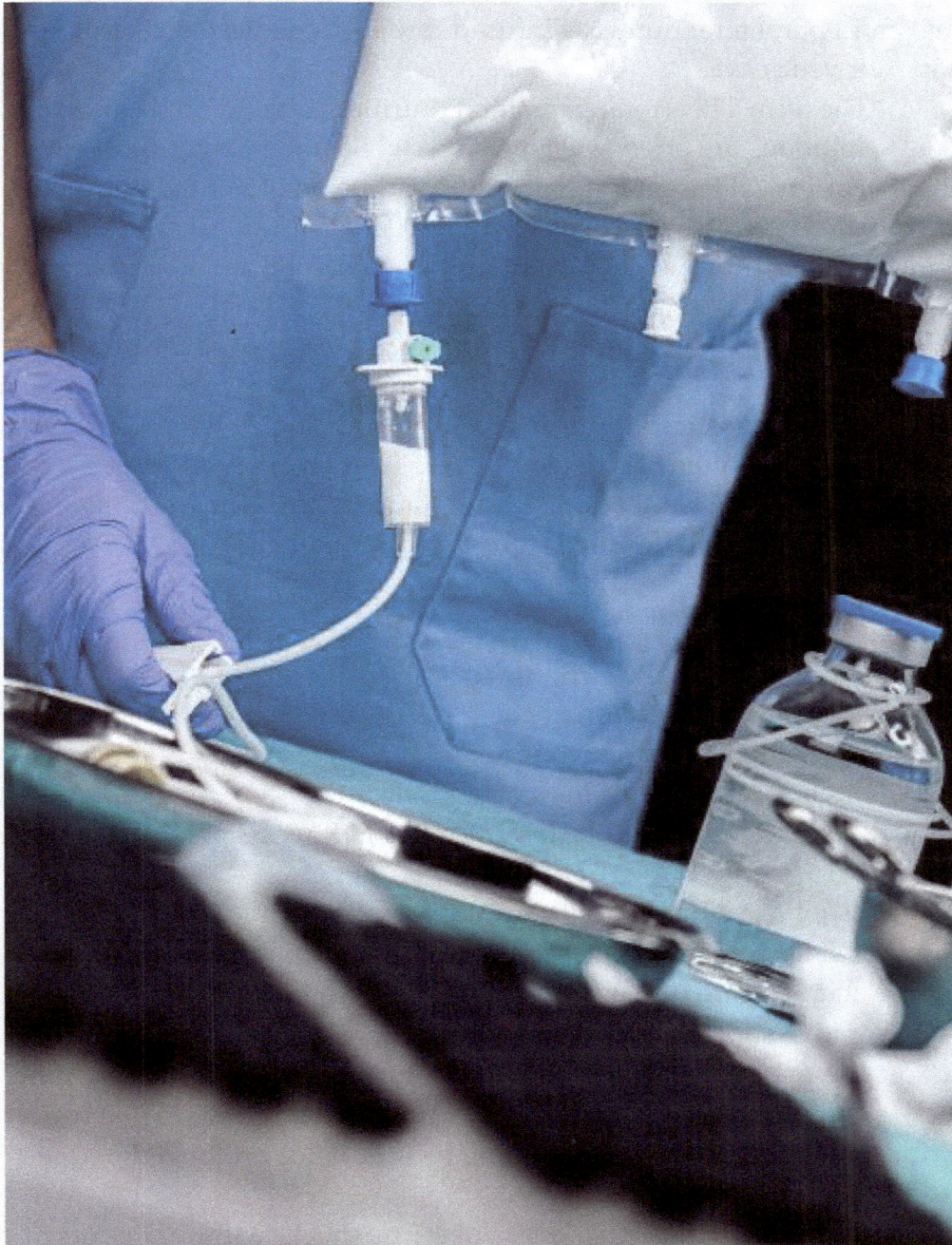

PN INDICATIONS AND INITIATION

Definitions

- CPN = Central Parenteral Nutrition → infusion of hyperosmolar (>900 mOsm/L) parenteral nutrients infused through a dedicated central line into the superior vena cava
  - The term TPN (total parenteral nutrition) should not be used because solutions are often > 900 mOsm/L while not meeting 100% (total) needs
- PPN = Peripheral Parenteral Nutrition → infusion of limited nutrients through peripheral IV access (max osmolarity < 900 mOsm/L)
- 3-in-1 TNA = Total Nutrient Admixture → dextrose, amino acids, and lipids compounded in 1 homogeneous solution
- 2-in-1 → dextrose and amino acid solution; lipids may be infused via Y connection
- ILE = Intravenous Lipid Emulsion; available as single oil (SO), usually soy, or mixed oil (MO), often SMOF (soy/MCT/olive/fish oils)
- MCB-PN = Multi-Chamber Bag PN → standardized commercially available formulas that are safe for medically stable PN patients

PN Indications

- Severely diminished GI function
  - Severe Malabsorption
  - SBS with high ostomy output
  - SBO, paralytic ileus, mesenteric ischemia
- GI fistula – except when output < 200 ml or EN Access able to be obtained distal to or directly through fistula
- Severe esophageal disease with inability to obtain EN access
- Multiple failed attempts to feed enterally or to obtain EN access
- Severe acute necrotizing pancreatitis
- Perioperative support of patients with moderate to severe malnutrition
  - **In post-op patients with NPO status or EN intolerance, wound healing may be impaired if PN not started within 5-10 days** `New`
- Critical illness who will have nothing by mouth for prolonged periods
- Additional Considerations:
  - Avoid PN in the acute phase of septic shock (within 24 hours of onset)
  - Trial prokinetic agents and/or post-pyloric access prior to initiating PN
  - Refusal of feeding tube is NOT an appropriate indication for PN
  - Central PN is preferred for PN > 7-14 days

PN Initiation Timing

Low Nutrition Risk	NPO > 7 days when EN not feasible
High Nutrition Risk Severe Malnutrition	PN as soon as feasible when po/EN not feasible - benefit in both moderate & severe PCM
Supplemental PN Use	Unable to meet >60% needs via EN for > 7 days
PN Discontinuation	Once EN/po intake tolerated at > 60% estimated needs

- **Patients of low nutrition risk/no malnutrition, PN <u>can be</u> delayed up to 7 days**
- **Maximal benefit is derived in severely malnourished patients who receive PN for more than 7-10 days**
- Consider PN when EN cannot be initiated for ≥ 7 days

> **New studies have found no difference in clinical outcomes between EN & PN in critically ill patients**

- **Avoid PN during acute phase of septic shock**
- PN should only be initiated in patients who are hemodynamically stable and who can tolerate the fluid volume and protein, CHO and ILE doses necessary to provide adequate nutrient substrate
- Patients whose PN is managed by an interdisciplinary team have significantly reduced metabolic fluid, and electrolyte complications as compared with patients managed by individual clinicians
- PN formulations are hypertonic to body fluids and, if administered inappropriately, may result in venous thrombosis, suppurative thrombophlebitis, or extravasation

Supplemental PN (SPN)

- Consider when unable to meet > 60% needs for > <u>7 days</u> per ASPEN
  - ESPEN recommends within 4-7 days
- Patients likely to benefit from SPN: polytrauma, open abdomen, frequent OR needs, ECMO, persistent hemodynamic instability, severe TBI, SAH with frequent vasospasm monitoring, repeat I&D/VAC changes

NUTRITION SUPPORT INITIATION

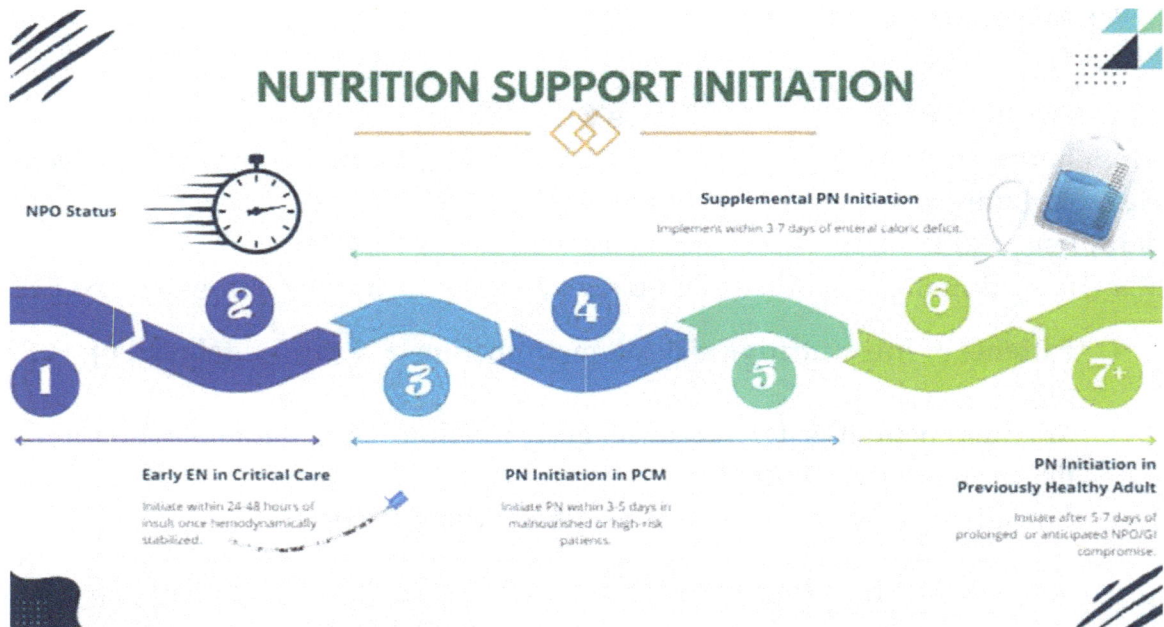

NPO Status

Supplemental PN Initiation
Implement within 3-7 days of enteral caloric deficit.

Early EN in Critical Care
Initiate within 24-48 hours of insult once hemodynamically stabilized.

PN Initiation in PCM
Initiate PN within 3-5 days in malnourished or high-risk patients.

PN Initiation in Previously Healthy Adult
Initiate after 5-7 days of prolonged or anticipated NPO/GI compromise.

PN Formulations

- Maximum volume recommended = 4L, free fluid from sterile water
- CHO source is dextrose, which provides 3.4 kcal/g
    - Dosage range = 150-450 g/day
    - Available in 50-70% concentrations
    - Final concentration for PN stability should be > 10-25%
    - Rare corn allergy hypersensitivity possible
- PRO generally assumed to be 16% nitrogen (6.25 g AA = 1 g nitrogen), includes essential & non-essential AAs; provides 4 kcal/g
    - Available in 10-20% concentrations
    - Special AA formulations not available
    - Some formulations also contain electrolytes
    - Crystalline nature of AA solutions impacts pH & formula stability
        - Basic nature of AA solutions improves lipid stability in TNA
        - Preferred: Aminosyn II, Travasol, Prosol, Clinosol (pH 5.8-7)
        - 15-20% concentrated solutions (Plenamine) and pediatric/neonatal solutions have marginal pH of 5.4-5.7
    - Protein provided in IV amino acid mixture is 17% less than assumed
        - For example: to provide 1-1.5 g/pro via PN, need to administer 1.2-1.8 g of a mixed AA solution

- Lipids: provides 10 kcal/g (vs 9) due to glycerol backbone
    - SO (soy) & Clinolipid (soy & olive oils) available in 20-30% concentrations
    - MO-SMOF available in 10-20-30% concentrations, providing 1.1, 2, 2.9 kcal/g respectively
    - 30% ILE only approved for use in TNA
    - Daily lipid dose should not exceed 60% of total energy or 2.5g/kg/day
    - SMOF mean essential FA concentrations: 35 mg/ML linoleic acid & 4.5mg/ML α-linolenic acid
        - Recommended 2-4% total concentration to meet EFA needs
        - Egg phospholipid emulsifier in SMOF = 15 mmol phosphate/liter
        - MCT source is coconut oil
        - Watch for allergens – soy, egg, fish, peanuts (cross-reaction)
    - Max lipid infusion rate: < 0.11 g/kg/hr
    - ASPEN recommendations for critical care patients- withhold soybean-based ILE or limit to a maximum of 200 g in 2 doses during first week if at risk of EFAD
    - Presence of MCT improves stability of ILE
    - Fat overload syndrome can occur if lipid infusion rate > clearance rate
        - Symptoms: headaches, seizure, fevers, jaundice, abdominal pain, hepatosplenomegaly, pancytopenia, ARDS, shock

PN Access

TPN usually hyperosmolar (1300-1800 mOsm/L)

Osmolarity		
Dextrose	5 mOsm/g	
Protein	10 mOsm/g	
Electrolytes	1-2 mOsm/mEq of each electrolyte additive	

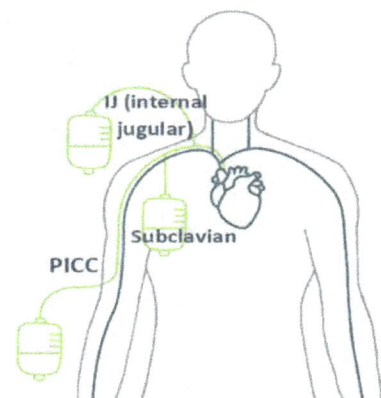

Peripheral Parenteral Nutrition (PPN)

- Maximum Dextrose: 150-300 g/d, AA: 50-100 g/d; Lipids unrestricted
- Can Y in separate lipids, but be cautious of osmolarity
- Electrolyte limitations: max 40 mEq/l K+; max 5 mEq/L calcium
- **Maximum osmolarity tolerated by a peripheral vein is 900 mOsm/L**
- May cause phlebitis and frequent (Q48-72 hr) IV site rotation
    - Heparin, small amounts of hydrocortisone, or nitro paste at insertion site may help prevent thrombophlebitis

- PPN Limitations:
  - ✓ Short-term therapy up to 2 weeks
  - ✓ Must have good peripheral venous access to avoid thrombophlebitis or extravasation injury
  - ✓ Should be able to tolerate large volumes of fluids (2.5-3 L/d)
  - ✓ Cannot meet high nutrient needs
- Midline catheters are recommended for PPN > 6 days due to longer catheter length and decreased likelihood of dislodging
  - o Tip no further than the axillary vein
  - o Can remain in for 2-6 weeks
  - o **Safe for PPN formulations only**

Central PN

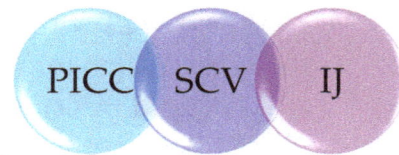

- Commonly referred to as TPN (total parenteral nutrition), though best practice is to describe access route and identify as central PN support
- PN requires a dedicated catheter lumen
- The SVC (superior vena cava) is the preferred vessel for central access for rapid dilution of PN solutions that are hypertonic with > 900 mOsm/L
- Repeated use of SCV is associated with risk of stenosis which is problematic for renal patients who require AV fistulas or shunts for hemodialysis
  - o Nephrologists should be consulted before PICC insertion
  - o Right IJ is the most direct approach to SVC for patients with CKD who may require dialysis
- Tunneled Central Catheters – Safe and effective for therapies ranging from months to years
- Implanted ports have the lowest rates of CRBSI in cancer patients
- Catheter Insertion – Requires the application of care bundle guidelines, hand hygiene, skin antisepsis using 0.5% chlorhexidine in alcohol solution, max sterile barrier precautions, and selection of appropriate venous access
- Care of the catheter exit site and hub critical to decrease the risk for CRS
  - o CDC guidelines recommend skin prep with >0.5% CHG preparation containing alcohol
- Flushing volume should be twice the volume of the catheter
- Antiseptic lock solutions include ethanol, taurolidine, citrate, 26% sodium chloride, and EDTA
  - o CVADs made of polyurethane material have ruptured and split with ethanol locks, but safe for use with silicone catheters

BASELINE ASSESSMENT

🕐   Indication required & anticipated duration as able

🍴   Consult RD for macronutrient recommendations & assistance with management

⚖️   Accurate weight, height, BMI   -Dry weight if volume overloaded
                                            -Prepregnancy weight for hyperemesis
                                            gravidarum patients

🧑   Baseline Labs: CMP, Mg, Phos, Alb, PAB, TGs, LFTs

Macronutrients

Protein

- Provides 4 kcal/g
- Maintenance: 1.0-1.3 g/kg
- Repletion, Surgery, Wounds: Start at 1.5 g/kg
- Can start at goal in TPN provided adequate renal function
- Generally assumed to be 16% nitrogen (6.25 g AA = 1 g nitrogen), includes essential & non-essential AAs
- Standard 10% AA solution (ex Aminosyn, TrophAmine, Freeamine)
    - Contains 10 mmol NaPhos per 100g protein & 89 mEq acetate/L
- 15% AA solution (ex Plenamine) more appropriate if volume restriction needed
    - Contains 3-5% more BCAA, no significant Phos, 147 mEq acetate/L

Dextrose

- Provides 3.4 kcal/g
- Available in 50-70% concentrations
- Recommended for 60-70% of nonprotein kcal
- Start at 100g or 50% goal (whichever is less) and advance by 1/3 goal daily if refeeding risk
    - If getting 120g in dextrose-containing IVF, ok to start at 120-150g in TPN

Parenteral Lipids

- Provides 10 kcal/g (includes glycerol backbone)
- 30-40% of nonprotein kcal
- Hold IL for TG > 400
- Standard ILEs are soy-based & proinflammatory
  - Indicated for short-term use
- Daily lipid dose should not exceed 60% of total energy or 2.5g/kg/day
- ILEs are oil-in-water emulsions consisting of 1 or more TG-containing oils, glycerin, and a phospholipid emulsifier
- Lipids are iso-osmolar & alkaline in nature (pH = 9)
- Commercial parenteral ILE available in TG concentrations of 10%, 20%, 30%
  - Avoid using 10% due to high phospholipid to triglyceride content
    - Propofol is a 10% solution
- Currently approved ILEs in US:
  - Intralipid or Nutrilipid – 20% soy-based SO-ILE (single-oil)
  - Clinolipid – 20% MO-ILE containing soy & olive oils (mixed oil)
  - SMOF – 20% MO-ILE containing soy, MCT, olive oil, fish oil
  - Omegaven – 10% fish oil-based SO-ILE *(approved only in Peds)*
- Parenteral ILEs are structurally designed so the chylomicron-like particles (micelles) within each emulsion resemble natural chylomicrons with respect to size, core TG and a layer of phospholipid
- SMOF lipids available for select patient populations
  - SMOF mean essential FA concentrations: 35 mg/ML linoleic acid & 4.5mg/ML α-linolenic acid
  - Egg phospholipid emulsifier in SMOF = 15 mmol phosphate per liter
- ASPEN recommendations for critical care patients- withhold soybean-based ILE or limit to a max of 200 g in 2 doses during first week if at risk of EFAD

EFA Supplementation in Critical Illness (ASPEN/SCCM guidelines)

- Avoid the routine use of all specialty formulas in critically ill patients in a medical ICU and all disease-specific formulas in the surgical ICU
- Immune-modulating formulas should not be routinely used in the medical ICU
- No recommendation can currently be made regarding anti-inflammatory enteral products in patients with ARDS or severe lung injury
- Formulations that contain fish oil and arginine can be _considered_ (_weak recommendation_) in severe trauma patients or patients with TBIs
  - Newer studies show decreased infection rate but longer vent days & ICU length of stay **Change**
- Immune-modulating formulas are recommended to be routinely used in the surgical ICU in postoperative patients requiring EN – _this rec holds up_
- New meta-analysis shows that α-3 supplementation doesn't decrease cardiovascular mortality risk, but actual fish intake does
  - Exception: 4 g/day α-3 supplement containing EPA or EPA + DHA can decrease CV & atherosclerosis risk in hypertriglyceridemia

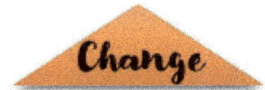

SMOF Lipids

- Indications
  - Long-term PN > 2 weeks
  - LFTs > 3x normal values
  - Critically Ill Patients
  - Severe Malnutrition
- Additional Considerations
  - Contains olive oil, soybean oil, MCT, and fish oil to provide healthy balance of dietary fats
  - Less omega-6 that standard soybean oil infusions – may need ↑ dose

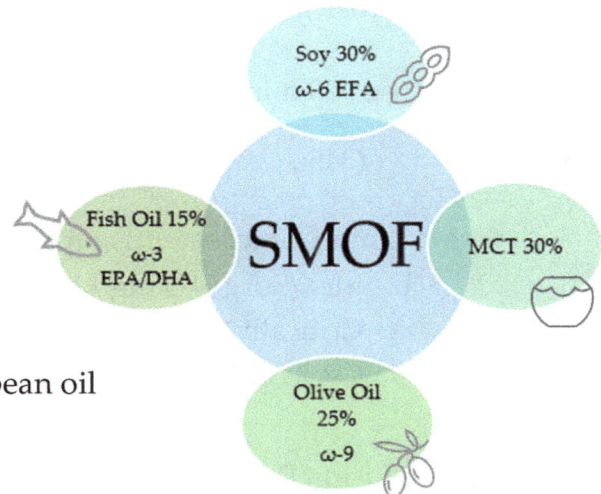

Soy 30%
ω-6 EFA

Fish Oil 15%
ω-3
EPA/DHA

SMOF

MCT 30%

Olive Oil 25%
ω-9

Sample PN Calculation

Based on needs assessed at 2000 kcal (25/kg) with 80g protein (1.0/kg) for wt 80 kg.

<u>PN Macronutrient Calculations:</u> *AA = 4 kcal/g, dextrose = 3.4 kcal/g, lipids = 10 kcal/g*

AA: 80 grams (320 kcal)

Nonprotein kcal: 1680 kcal (2000 total- 320 protein)
Assuming 70/30 dextrose/lipids

Dextrose
- 70% of 1680 = 1175 kcal dextrose / 3.4 g/kcal = 345 grams dex

Lipids
- 30% of 1680 = 500 kcal lipid/ 10 g/kg = 50 grams lipid

Recommendation = **80g AA, 345 g dex, 50 g lipid**

<u>Glucose Infusion Rate:</u>
Max dextrose infusion rate: 4-5 mg/kg/min continuous; < 7 mg/kg/min for cycled PN
Dextrose mg/kg/min for a 24-hr infusion:
dextrose g/day x 1000 (to convert to mg) / 1440 (60 min/hr x 24 hrs) / wt =
mg/kg/min
(use 720 min for 12 hr cycle, 840 for 14 hr cycle, or 1080 for 16 hr cycle)

(345g dextrose x 1000) / 1440 min / 80 kg = **2.99 mg/kg/min**

- Maximum Glucose Infusion Rates:
    - Med/Surg: 4-5 mg/kg/minute
    - Critically Ill: < 4 mg/kg/minute
    - Cycled PN: < 7 mg/kg/minute at peak infusion

<u>Lipid Infusion Rate:</u> *Max lipid infusion rate: 0.11 g/kg/hr*

Lipid g/kg/hr for 24-hr infusion:
Lipid g/day / wt (kg) / 24 hrs

50 g lipid / 80 kg / 24 hrs = **0.026 g/kg/hr**

PN Volume Calculations:

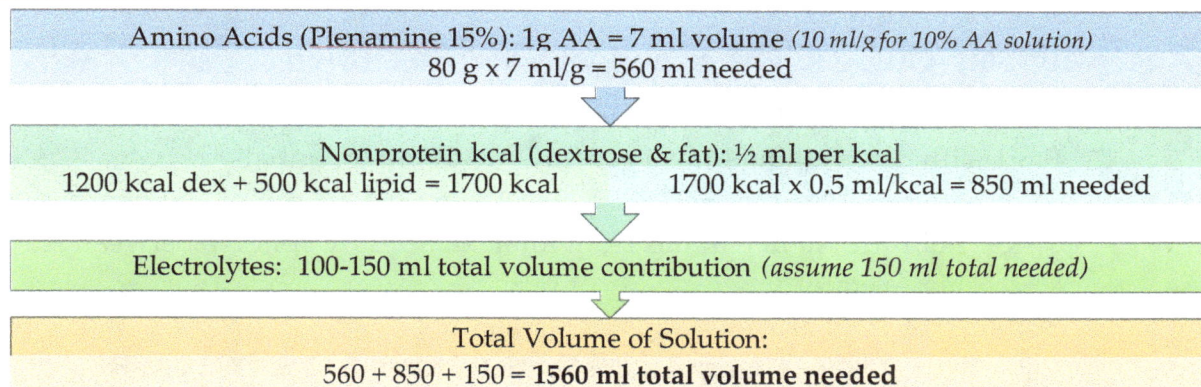

Amino Acids (Plenamine 15%): 1g AA = 7 ml volume *(10 ml/g for 10% AA solution)* 80 g x 7 ml/g = 560 ml needed

⬇

Nonprotein kcal (dextrose & fat): ½ ml per kcal
1200 kcal dex + 500 kcal lipid = 1700 kcal   1700 kcal x 0.5 ml/kcal = 850 ml needed

⬇

Electrolytes: 100-150 ml total volume contribution *(assume 150 ml total needed)*

⬇

Total Volume of Solution: 560 + 850 + 150 = **1560 ml total volume needed**

Volume Considerations

- Patients may be limited on volume for many reasons, such as impaired renal function, heart failure, volume overload w/ respiratory compromise, elderly patients
- Protein contributes greatest volume & osmolarity
- Volume Concentration
  - Amino Acids
    - 15% solution: 1g AA = 7 ml volume
    - 20% solution: 1g AA = 10 ml volume
  - Nonprotein kcal (dextrose & fat)
    - 2-in-1: g dextrose/70% solution = ml fluid needed
    - 3-in-1 TNA: need 0.5 ml/kcal dextrose + lipids
  - Need 100-200 ml for micronutrients + additives

Osmolarity

Dextrose	5 mOsm/g
Protein	10 mOsm/g
Electrolytes	1-2 mOsm/mEq of each electrolyte additive

Na and K contribute roughly 2 mOsm/mEq, Ca about 1.4 mOsm/mEq, and Mg about 1 mOsm/mEq.

> ### Sample Osmolarity Calculation:
>
> 1. 150 g dextrose x 5 mOsm/g = 750 mOsm
> 2. 50 g AA x 10 mOsm/g = 500 mOsm
> 3. 150 mEq of electrolytes x 1 mOsm/mEq = 150 mOsm
> 4. 750 + 500 + 150 = **1400 mOsm**

Electrolytes and Additives

Step-By-Step Guide to Ordering Initial PN Electrolytes:

1. Volume determination –start with current IVF volume
2. Start with determining Phos –generally 10-20 mmol initially
   - 20 mmol NaPhos = 27 mEq Na (1.33 mEq Na/1 mmol NaPhos)
   - Subtract Na in NaPhos from total Na needs & split Na between NaCl & Na Acetate
3. Sodium can start at 2 mEq/kg or equivalent of ½ NS
   - Start at 50/50 split and adjust based on serum Cl & CO_2 levels
   - Replace base deficit with acetate; generally, add 10mEq acetate per 1 mm/L CO_2 < 24
4. Target serum K+ level of 4.0
   - 10 mEq of KCl needed to increase serum K+ by 0.1 mg/dL
   - Start K+ conservatively ~ 20-40 mEq – safer to replete with riders
5. Mg & Calcium can start at low end of above ranges & adjust as needed

---

Additional Notes:

SMOF contains 15 mmol Phos/L

1 mmol IV K^+Phos = 1.47 mEq K^+

1 mmol IV Na Phos = 1.33 mEq Na

10% AA contains 10 mmol NaPhos per 100g protein & 89 mEq acetate/L

15% AA contains 147 mEq acetate/L, no significant Phos

Electrolyte Management

Element	Reference Range	PN Provision	Available Preparations	Considerations
Na	136 – 144	1 – 2 mEq/kg	NaCl Na Acetate Na Phos	↑ needs w/ GI losses
K	3.6 – 5.1	1 – 2 mEq/kg	KCl K Acetate K Phos	↑ needs w/ GI losses, refeeding, meds
Chloride	101 – 111	PRN to maintain acid/base balance	NaCl KCl	↑ needs w/ metabolic alkalosis, volume depletion
Acetate	CO_2 22 -29	PRN to maintain acid/base balance	Na Acetate K Acetate	↑ needs w/ renal failure, metabolic acidosis, bicarb GI losses
Phos	2.4 – 4.7	10 – 40 mmol/day	Na Phos K Phos	↑ needs w/ high dextrose loads, refeeding
Mg	1.8 – 2.5	8 – 20 mEq/day	Mg Sulfate	↑ needs w/ GI losses, drugs, refeeding
Calcium*	8.9 – 10.3	10 – 15 mEq/day	Ca gluconate	↑ needs w/ high protein intake

*Corrected Ca (mg/dL) = Measured Ca (mg/dL) + 0.8 [4 – serum albumin (g/dL)]

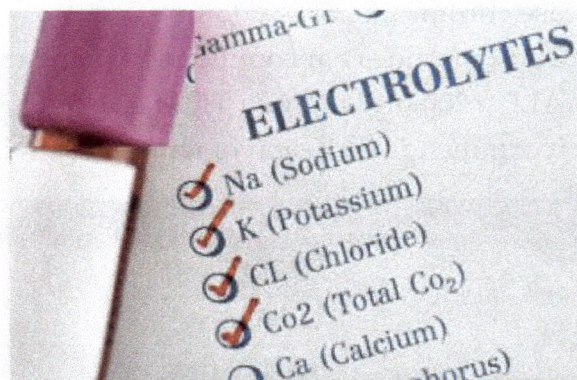

Parenteral Vitamins

- Include ascorbic acid, retinol, ergocalciferol or cholecalciferol, thiamine, riboflavin, pyridoxine, niacinamide, dexpanthenol, dl-α tocopheryl acetate, folic acid, cyanocobalamin, biotin, phyntonadione
- Addition of Vitamin K creates concern for those who are on anticoagulation to maintain patency of devices
- Vitamin D preparations are challenging because high-dose parenteral formulas of Vitamin D are unavailable in the US

Vitamin	Standard Daily Requirement	Vitamin	Standard Daily Requirement
Thiamine (B₁)	6 mg	Biotin	60 mcg
Riboflavin (B₂)	3.6 mg	Ascorbic Acid	200 mg
Niacin (B₃)	40 mg	Vitamin A	990 mcg
Folic Acid	600 mcg	Vitamin D	5 mcg
Pantothenic Acid	15 mg	Vitamin E	10 mg
Pyridoxine (B₆)	6 mg	Vitamin K	150 mcg
Cyanocobalamin (B₁₂)	5 mcg		

Parenteral Trace Elements (TE)

- Published recommendations for daily parenteral intake of zinc, copper, manganese, and chromium as well as selenium supplementation
- **ILE is disrupted by iron, so iron dextran can only be added to 2-in-1 formulas**
- Zinc: Usual supplemental dose 3-5 mg. Increased needs in patients with consistent high GI losses. Start 3 mg/day.
- Hold selenium if impaired renal function
- May need to decrease chromium in renal failure
- Current TE formulation provides > recommended manganese & copper
- If T bili $\geq$ 3 and/or ALP > 200 mg/dL, hold TE & give 5mg Zn + 60 mcg Se
- ASPEN no longer recommends inclusion of chromium in PN TE

Trace Element	Standard Daily Requirement
Copper	0.3-0.5 mg
Manganese	55 mcg
Selenium	60-100 mcg
Zinc	3-5 mg

US TE Product Composition:

TE (1 ml)	Multrys™ Neonates/Peds < 10kg	Tralement™ Peds/Adults > 10 kg
Zinc	1000 mcg	3 mg
Copper	50 mcg	0.3 mg
Manganese	3 mcg	55 mcg
Selenium	6 mcg	60 mcg

Carnitine

- Necessary for proper transport & metabolism of LCFA into matrix of mitochondria for beta oxidation
  - Carnitine deficiency → impaired fatty acid oxidation → hepatic stenosis
  - Supplemental dose: 200 mg/mL L-carnitine
  - Neonates and infants are more susceptible to carnitine deficiency

Micronutrient Dosing

- Multivitamins (MVI): 10 ml/day
- Trace Elements (TE): 1 ml/day
  - If need to hold Cu & Mn, add extra 3 mg zinc & 60 mcg selenium
- Supplemental Zinc: 3-5 mg/day
  - Increased needs in patients with consistent high GI losses.
- Supplemental Thiamine: 100-300 mg/day
  - Indicated for malnutrition/refeeding risk, hx bariatric sx, ETOH abuse

Medications should not be added to PN unless evidence of stability, compatibility, and therapeutic efficacy
- Octreotide in PN loses effective drug activity

PN Component Shortages

- *See ASPEN website for timely recommendations (nutritioncare.org)*
- If requires PN longer than 2 weeks, should receive a total of 100 g of soybean oil-based ILE per week to avoid EFAD
- Ration or Reserve IV MVI or TE for patients solely on PN or those with therapeutic needs
- Consider using oral or enteral MVI or TE preparations if tolerated
- Administer individual parenteral trace entities once out of multi-trace products

Multiple Chamber Bag PN (MCB-PN)

- Commercial PN formulations, "starter PN"
- Usually lower cost and less risk of compounding errors
- Can be used for PPN or CPN, depending on osmolarity
- Limit to 1L for initial PPN if concern for fluid overload or poor vasculature
- Available as 2 (ex Clinimix) or 3 chamber (ex Kabiven/Perikabiven) bags
  - Baxter: 2-in-1 CPN & PPN options
    - CLINIMIX® - no electrolytes
    - CLINIMIX-E®- with electrolytes
    - Can be piggy-backed with IV lipid emulsions
  - Fresenius Kabi: 3-in-1 CPN & PPN options with electrolytes
    - KABIVEN® - central PN only
    - PERIKABIVEN® - CPN or PPN
- Chamber activation required to mix into homogenous solution
- MVI & TE must be added prior to administration
- Lipids need to Y in separately
  - Standard stock solutions for lipids come in 10% or 20% solution in 250 mL or 500 mL bags

2 Chamber	3 Chamber
• Lipids Y in separately • Can use SO-ILE or MO-ILE • Available with or without electrolytes so able to customize based on manufacturer compatibility	○ **SO-ILE is the only available lipid formulation in 3 chamber MCB** ○ Fixed electrolyte contents

Electrolyte Considerations:

- Often contain more Cl- salts, which affects pH & compatibility
- Electrolytes are listed on labels in ion form, not salt form or concentration per liter or per bag as required for compounded PN
- Electrolyte-free solution has greater ability to customize added electrolytes, either compounded by Pharmacy or in form of riders
- Electrolyte-containing solutions may need to be limited volume in CKD
- Standard electrolytes may not meet needs in refeeding syndrome

Additional Considerations:

- If wasting a partial bag, additives are lost proportionally
- Higher needs will require CPN & higher volume

COMPOUNDING PN

- Common bulk products
  - AA: 10%, 15%, or 20% concentrations
  - Dextrose: 30%, 50%, or 70% concentrations
  - 20% ILE available for TNA or direct administration
  - 30% SO-ILE available for TNA only
  - To calculate, start with volume of component x % concentration/ 100

PN Compounding & Stock Solution Calculations

> Patient is receiving 250 ml of 70% dextrose, 250 ml of 20% ILE and 10% AA solution providing 100g protein.
> Calculate total energy and volume requirements.

Energy Calculation

Have grams protein, need to calculate dextrose & lipid:

- Dextrose = 250 ml x 0.7 (70%) = 175g dextrose in solution
  x 3.4 kcal/g = 595 kcal dextrose
- Lipids = 250 ml x 0.2 (20%) = 50g lipid
  x 10 kcal/g = 500 kcal lipid
- Protein = 100g x 4 kcal/g = 400 kcal
  So, for kcal provision, 595 + 500 + 400 = **1495 kcal**

Volume Calculation

Have volume dextrose & lipid, need to calculate protein:

- Protein requires 10 ml volume/g protein in a 10% solution,
  so 100g x 10 ml/g = 1000 mL
  So, for total volume, 1000 + 250 + 250 = **1500 ml**

Additional Example:

Patient is receiving 500 ml of 60% dextrose, 250 ml of 20% ILE & 10% AA solution providing 90g protein

- Dextrose: 500 ml x 0.6 = 300 grams x 3.4 kcal/g = 1020 kcal
- Lipid: 250 ml x 0.2 = 50 grams x 10 kcal/g kcal = 500 kcal
- Protein: 90 x 4 kcal/g = 360 kcal
  - 90g x 10 ml/g = 900 ml volume need
- Total kcal provided: 1020 + 500 + 360 = 1880 kcal
- Total volume needed before electrolytes: 500 + 250 + 900 = 1650 ml

PN STABILITY, LABELING, & SAFETY

Formulation Stability

- Most instability is associated with the addition of ILEs or MVIs
  - Add MVI last, shortly before administration, never to ILE alone
- Other causes of instability: pH, temperature, light, O_2, solvents or reactants
- Final concentration of AAs > 4% and IVFEs > 2-2.5% to improve stability
  - Low AA content reduces buffering capacity of TPN solution
  - ILE of 1% might be stable enough with AA > 5%
- Electrolytes: Ca ≤ 10/L; Phos ≤ 30/L; K & Na ≤ 200/L
  - Excess cation amounts (Mg & Ca) can reduce stability in 3-in-1
    - Keep Ca + Mg ≤ 20/L
  - Excess Ca & Phos can cause micro-precipitates
    - Compounding should add Phos first & Ca last

45 rule Ca + (2x Phos) ≤ 45/L   **200 rule** Ca x Phos ≤ 200/L

- Some aluminum contamination in TE is common – should be < 5 mcg/kg/day
  - Max permitted is 25 mcg/L
- Renal Considerations: doses of K^+, Phos, Mg, Ca^{2+} should be decreased by 50%
- Acid-Base Balance: Dextrose (pH 3.5-5.5) < Amino Acids < Lipids (pH 9)
  - For every 0.1 decrease in pH, potassium will rise by 0.6 mEq/L
  - For every 0.1 increase in pH, potassium will decrease by 0.6 mEq/L

Use of Filters

- Needed to prevent Ca+ Phos precipitation
- Large pore filters needed- (5μm) to remove precipitates, particulate matter, pathogenic microorganisms
- Lipid particles > 5 μm can cause fat embolism
  - Symptoms; hypotension, pulmonary hypertension, acidosis
- Filter limitations: fat droplets-need to use 1.2μm filters with TNA PN formulas
- A 0.22μm filter should be used for dextrose amino acid PN or 2-in-1

3-in-1 1.2 μm filter Place near catheter hub Change Q24h

2-in-1 0.22 μm filter Place below Y site when mixed w/ ILE Change Q12h

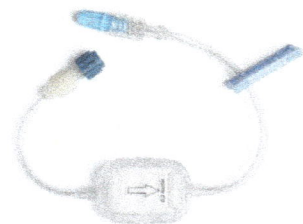

PN Safety

- **PN is a high alert medication**
- USP (United States Pharmacopeia) Chapter {797} safety guidelines:
  - PN BUD (beyond use date): 30 hours a continuous room temperature
  - Refrigerate up to 10 days, temp 2-8 °C
  - ASPEN has a Safe Practice Checklist available
- All products must use non-PVC materials
- Pharmacy should always complete a 2nd check of PN order and formulation
  - Pharmacist should visually inspect all CSP for physical deficit (ex TNA phase separation) and package integrity (ex leakage or improper seal)
- ASPEN PN Safety Consensus Recommendations for labeling:
  - Compounded macronutrient content should be listed in grams per 24-hr nutrient infusion to avoid misinterpretation
  - Electrolytes ordered as complete salt form rather than individual ion
  - Full generic name for each ingredient (*unless brand name can identify unique properties of specific dosage form*)

Label Requirements

- Patient identifiers & date of birth
- Height & dosing weight in metric units
- Allergies
- Diagnosis/diagnoses & indication(s) for PN
- Administration route/vascular access device
- Contact information for prescriber
- Date & time order submitted
- Administration date & time
- Volume, infusion rate, continuous vs cyclic
- Type of formulation (3-in-1 or 2-in-1)

Allergies

Component	Allergen/Reaction Risk
IV Dextrose	Corn
Intralipid	Soybean, egg; risk of cross-contamination with peanut
SMOF Lipid	Soybean, egg, fish; risk of cross-contamination with peanut
AA Solutions	Contraindicated in PKU so includes warning associated with aspartame allergy
IV Potassium	Latex reaction
IV Calcium	Can cause precipitate reaction with IV Ceftraxione (antibiotic)

2-in-1 or 3-in-1 Admixtures

- CDC recommends a 12-hr limit on hang time for separate ILE due to enhanced microbial growth potential
  - If needs continuous infusion, split into 2 doses with new tubing
- ILE incorporated into a TNA has a 24-hr hang time
- Creaming/aggregation of a TNA appears as a translucent band at the surface of the emulsion separate from the remaining TNA dispersion
  - Light creaming is common & not a concern for formula safety
- Cracking/oiling out can occur when pH of solution <5 or >10
  - These formulas are not safe for use and should be discarded
  - Ideal pH for lipid stability = 7-8
  - Low pH degrades the egg phospholipid emulsifier in ILEs

PN ADVANCEMENT & MANAGEMENT

Routine Monitoring

Daily	Weekly
Weight	PAB
BMP	TG
Mg	LFTs
Phos	(Hepatic Function
I/O's	Panel)

Cycling PN

- Ideally cycling should be a 2–3-day process by gradually condensing hours to prevent hyperglycemia
- Start w/ slow cycle for new TPN patients over 2-3 nights if hyperglycemic
- Need good BG control & volume tolerance to cycle over 10-12 hrs
- Max cycled GIR = 7 mg/kg/min
- Run at 50% rate for 1st & last hours to prevent hyper-/hypoglycemia

Electrolyte Renewal

	Too Low	Too High
Sodium	• Increase sodium • Consider decreasing fluid • Need 30-40 mEq Na to move level	• Increase fluid • Consider decreasing sodium
Chloride	• Increase Cl (preferably as NaCl) & decrease acetate as needed	• Decrease Cl & increase acetate as needed
Acetate	• Replace base deficit with acetate: add 10mEq acetate per 1 mm/L CO_2 < 24	• Decrease or hold acetate
Potassium	• Increase by 10 mEq for every 0.1 increase needed to reach target serum K^+ 4.0 • Include any KCl riders in mEq increase need calculation	• Decrease by 10 mEq for every 0.1 decrease needed to reach target serum K^+ 4.0 • Hold for K^+ > 5.0
Phosphorus	• Increase NaPhos in PN • If need > 25 mmol, add K^+Phos • If persistently low, check PTH level	• Decrease by 50% or hold • Add enteral phos binders if appropriate
Magnesium	• Each 1g (8 mEq) should ↑ serum Mg by 0.1 mg/dL – equilibrium takes up to 48 hours	• Decrease by 50% or hold
Calcium	• Add enteral phos binders as able if due to high Phos	• Decrease by 50% or hold

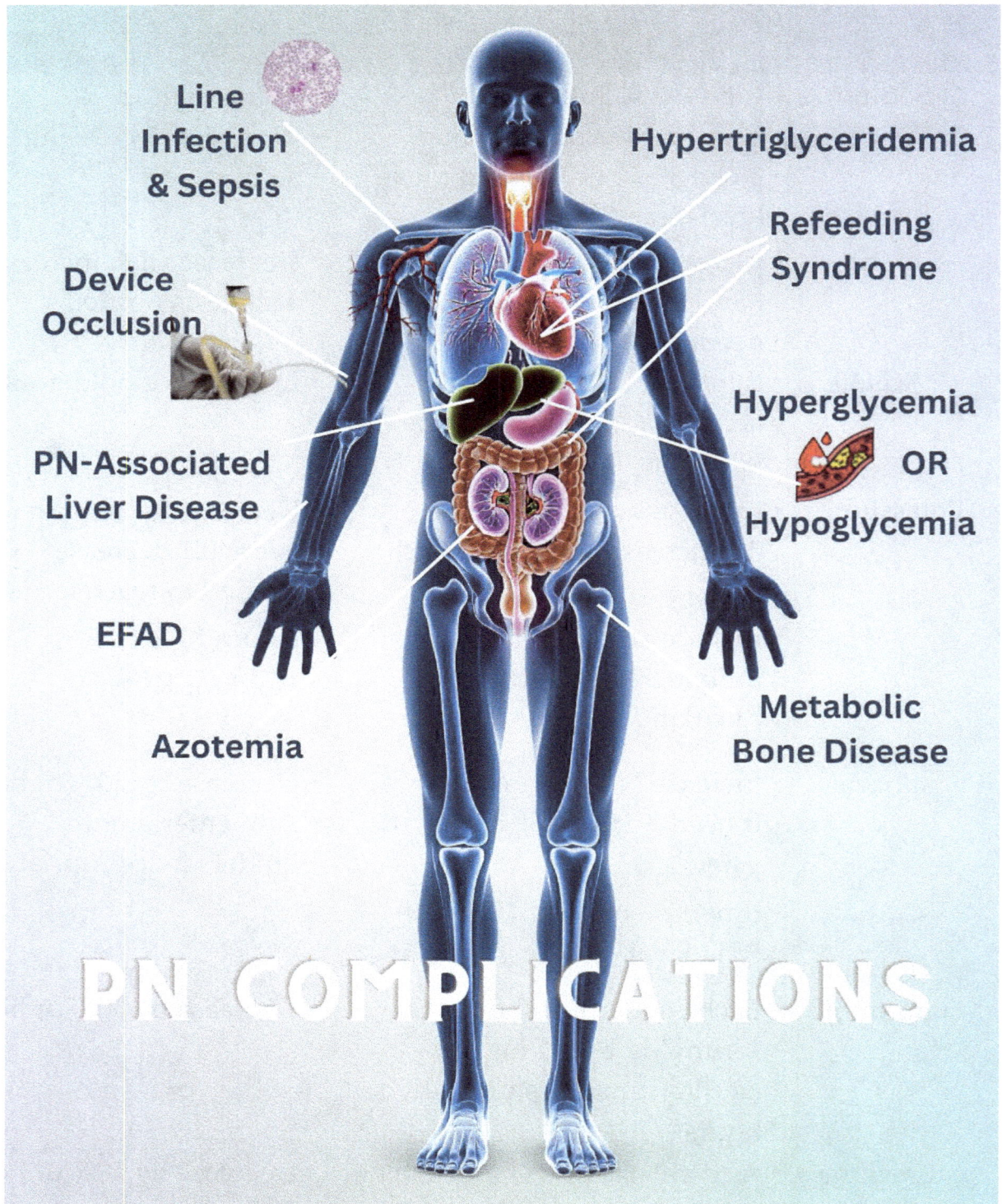

Line Infection & Sepsis

Hypertriglyceridemia

Device Occlusion

Refeeding Syndrome

PN-Associated Liver Disease

Hyperglycemia OR Hypoglycemia

EFAD

Azotemia

Metabolic Bone Disease

PN COMPLICATIONS

PN COMPLICATIONS

REFEEDING SYNDROME

- Refeeding Syndrome (RFS) is a metabolic & physiologic consequence of introducing nutrition, primarily carbohydrates, after a prolonged period of starvation.
- In the starved state, there is a total-body deficit of phosphorus, potassium, magnesium, and thiamine.
- When glucose appears in the bloodstream, insulin secretion rises in response, driving phosphorus and potassium intracellularly.
- The decrease in serum electrolytes may be sudden, severe, and deadly.

Presentation of Refeeding Syndrome (RFS)

ASPEN Definition: Any decrease in serum phosphorus, potassium, or magnesium within 5 days of initiating nutrition support.

Classification based on degree of electrolyte disturbances:

Mild	Moderate	Severe
10-20% decrease	20-30% decrease	>30% decrease

Serum Electrolyte Variability
- Serum electrolytes may appear normal initially despite intracellular depletion due to decrease in renal excretion to maintain serum homeostasis
- Phosphorus in particular often wnl prefeeding because cellular Phos is pulled into the bloodstream to maintain serum levels when intake deficient
- Sharpest decline often seen around days 2-3

Populations at Risk

Malnutrition	Failure to Thrive	AIDS	Cancer
Bariatric Surgery	Malabsorption Disorders	Major GI Surgery	Eating Disorders

Risk Stratification

	Moderate Risk 2 risk criteria needed	Significant Risk 1 risk criteria needed
BMI	16-18.5 kg/m²	< 16 kg/m²
Weight loss	5% in 1 month	7.5% in 3 months or > 10% in 6 months
Caloric intake	• None or negligible po for 5-6 days • <75% EER for > 7 days in acute illness • <75% EER for > 1 month	• None or negligible po for > 7 days • <50% EER for > 5 days in acute illness • <50% EER for > 1 month
Abnormal prefeeding serum Phos, K+, Mg	Minimally low levels	Moderate to significantly low levels
Loss of subcutaneous fat	Moderate loss	Severe loss
Loss of muscle mass	Mild to moderate loss	Severe loss
High-risk comorbidities	Moderate disease	Severe disease

Clinical Manifestations

ASPEN Consensus Recommendations
Prevention & Treatment of Refeeding Syndrome in Nutrition Support Patients

Initiation & Advancement of Calories:
- Initiate with 100-150g dextrose or 10-20 kcal/kg for first 24 hours; advance by 33% of goal every 1-2 days.
- Advance dextrose slowly to goal over 3-7 days.
- Hold initiation and advancement of calories in moderate- to high-risk patients until electrolytes are supplemented and stabilized.
- Delay initiation of nutrition support in patients with severely low phosphorus, potassium, or magnesium until levels corrected.

Vitamin Supplementation:
- Supplement thiamine in TPN – 100 mg/day prior to initiation of feeding and continue for minimum 5-7 days.
- MVI should be added to PN daily & supplemented for 10+ days for EN patients at risk of refeeding syndrome.

Monitoring:
- Monitor electrolytes every 12 hours for the first 3 days in high-risk patients & replete based on established standards of care.
- If electrolytes become more difficult to manage or drop precipitously during initiation of nutrition support, decrease to 50% caloric goal and resume advancement by 33% every 1-2 days.
- Check vital signs every 4 hours for first 24 hours in at-risk patients.
- Telemetry recommended for high-risk patients.

METABOLIC COMPLICATIONS

Essential Fatty Acid Deficiency

- EFAD symptoms: scaly dermatitis, alopecia, hepatomegaly, thrombocytopenia, fatty liver, anemia
- Triene: tetraene ratio >0.2 indicates EFAD and can occur within 1-3 weeks in adults receiving ILE-free PN

Hypertriglyceridemia

- Can occur with dextrose overfeeding or with rapid administration of ILE (>0.11g/kg/hr)
- Restrict to <30% of total energy or 1g/kg/day
- As separate infusion, give over at least 8-10 hours
- Hold or reduce ILE dose if serum TG >400 mL/dl (both Intralipid & SMOF)
- Pancreatitis due to ILE induced hypertriglyceridemia is rare unless TG >1000

Azotemia

- Excessive PRO administration ↑ the metabolic demand of disposing the byproducts of protein metabolism
- Patients with hepatic or renal disease are prone to development due to impaired metabolism and elimination of urea
- Hyperammonemia is a greater risk when protein hydrolysates contain excessive amounts of ammonia and insufficient arginine for urea cycle metabolism
- Rare occurrence since the advent of crystalline AA solutions except in patients with urea cycle defects
- Protein restriction in liver failure with hyperammonemia and encephalopathy is not associated with improved outcomes, so it is discouraged
- Use of high BCAA, low AAA formulations has inconsistent results and is not recommended
- Protein should not be restricted with AKI, CRRT, HD especially in malnourished patients

Trace Element Deficiency & Toxicity

- High intestinal losses can result in zinc deficiency
- Cardiomyopathy from selenium deficiency reported with long term PN without supplementation
- Toxicity potential with hepatobiliary disease – recommend remove copper and manganese

BLOOD GLUCOSE & INSULIN MANAGEMENT

Hyperglycemia

- Most common complication with PN and can be caused by various factors
- ASPEN recommends target BG concentration of 140-180 mg/dl in hospitalized adults receiving PN
- Initiate PN at ~150-200g for 1st 24 hours or ~100g/day with low BMI or poor glucose control
- Do not exceed 4-5mg/kg/min or 20-25 kcals/kg in acutely ill patients
- Initial insulin dose of 0.05-0.1 unit/g dextrose in PN solution or 0.15-0.2 units/g dextrose in those already with significant hyperglycemia; two-thirds of previous days requirement can be added to next day's PN bag

Hypoglycemia

- Hypoglycemia may occur with abrupt cessation of PN, regardless of whether the patient is receiving insulin, referred to as "rebound hypoglycemia"
- If the PN infusion must be interrupted, 10% dextrose in water infusion should be initiated at the same rate as the PN until PN infusion resumes
- To avoid rebound hypoglycemia associated with PN, taper the infusion during the last 1 to 2 hours prior to discontinuation

Intravenous Insulin Therapy

- During PN, many patients will require approximately double the insulin infusion rate over the level needed while NPO
- The insulin infusion rate should be decreased to the basal or NPO rate 30 to 60 minutes before the PN is discontinued to accommodate the gradual decrease in insulin provision

Estimation of the Total Daily Insulin Dose (TDD)

- For patients managed with IV insulin therapy, the total daily dose for subcutaneous insulin can be estimated as approximately 50% to 70% of the dose used IV to control blood glucose for 24 hours
- The clinician may use formulas based on body weight to estimate the total daily insulin dose

Type 1 DM	0.3 to 0.5 units/kg/d
Type 2 DM	0.5 to 0.8 units/kg/d
Very insulin-resistant T2 DM	0.9 to 1.5 units/kg/d
High-dose glucocorticoids	0.9 to 1.5 units/kg/d

- Total daily insulin dose can be estimated using the assumptions from the 1500 rule or the 1800 rule
  - 1500 Rule
    - estimates the sensitivity factor or the point drop in glucose (mg/dL) for every 1 unit of **regular** insulin
    - Ex: for TDD 60 units → 1500/60 = 25-point drop in BG (mg/dL)
  - 1800 Rule
    - estimates the sensitivity factor or the point drop in glucose (mg/dL) for every 1 unit of **rapid-acting** insulin (lispro, aspart)
    - Ex: for TDD 60 units → 1800/60 = 30-point drop in BG (mg/dL)

PN Insulin Calculations

- Initial: 0.05-0.1 units per gram dextrose if hyperglycemic and up to 0.2 units per gram if diabetic
  - Start calculations at low end of range in abundance of caution.
- Titration: add 1/2 to 2/3 total amount of sliding-scale insulin required over 24 hrs to next day's PN
- Max 0.3 units/gram dextrose or 100 units/day
- If persistent hyperglycemia with 0.3 units/gram of dextrose → basal or IV insulin needed

Sample Calculation

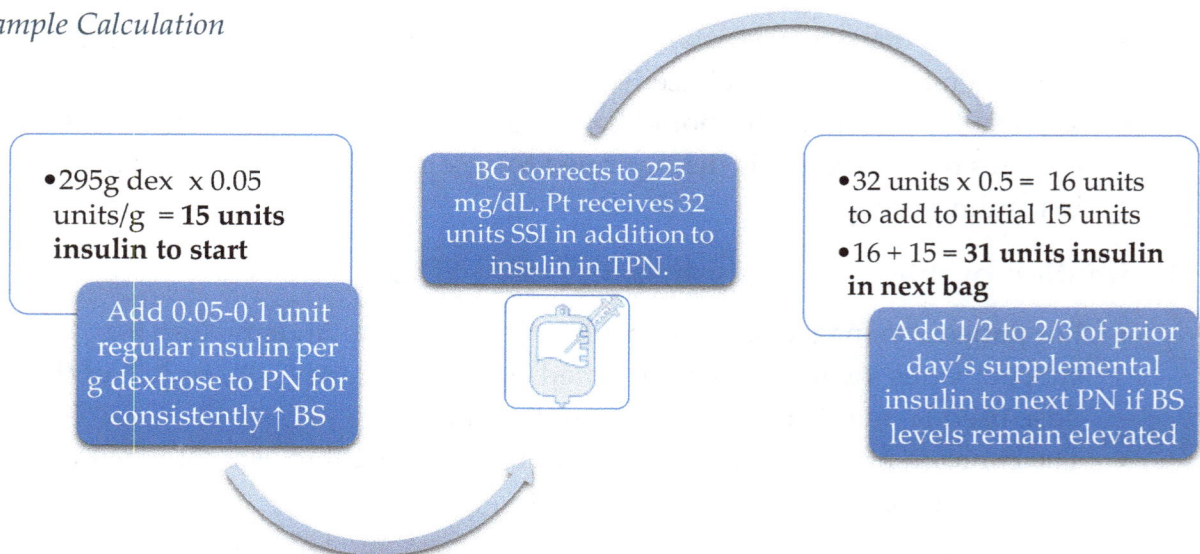

- 295g dex x 0.05 units/g = **15 units insulin to start**

  Add 0.05-0.1 unit regular insulin per g dextrose to PN for consistently ↑ BS

- BG corrects to 225 mg/dL. Pt receives 32 units SSI in addition to insulin in TPN.

- 32 units x 0.5 = 16 units to add to initial 15 units
- 16 + 15 = **31 units insulin in next bag**

  Add 1/2 to 2/3 of prior day's supplemental insulin to next PN if BS levels remain elevated

PN-ASSOCIATED LIVER DISEASE

- Steatosis – modest ↑ of serum aminotransferase concentration that occurs within 2 weeks of PN initiation & normalize when PN is discontinued. It can progress to fibrosis or cirrhosis in long-term PN patients
- Cholestasis (PNAC) is a condition of impaired secretion of bile or frank biliary obstruction that occurs primarily in children or long-term adult PN patients
    - Usually has elevated alkaline phosphatase, gamma-glutamyl transpeptidase (GGT), and conjugated (direct) bilirubin concentration with or without jaundice
    - Bilirubin >2 is considered the prime indicator for cholestasis
    - Serious as it can lead to cirrhosis and liver failure

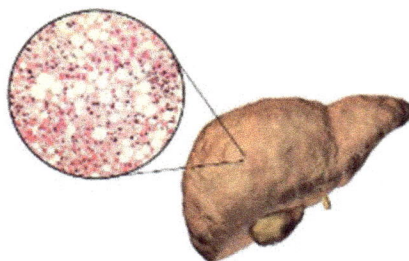

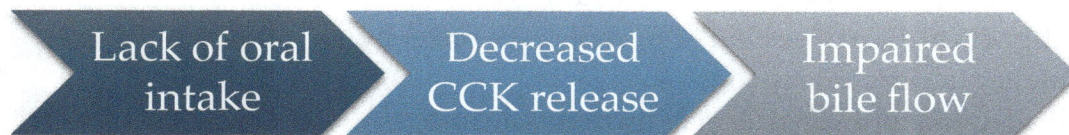

Lack of oral intake → Decreased CCK release → Impaired bile flow

- Gallbladder sludge/stones from gallbladder stasis can lead to cholecystitis
    - Duration on PN seems to correlate with development of biliary sludge
- Massive intestinal resection is a risk factor for PNALD
    - SB remnant <50cm has significant association with chronic cholestasis
- Chronic cholestasis and severe PNALD strongly associated with ILE intake >1g/kg/day in long term PN
- Carnitine – plays an important role in fat metabolism and when added to PN has been shown to help mobilize hepatic fat stores and prevent steatosis in neonates
    - No improvement found with adult liver enzymes despite normalization of serum carnitine concentrations
- PN modifications: remove copper & manganese, reduce dextrose, decrease ILE <1g/kg/day, cycle; initiate trophic EN/po as able

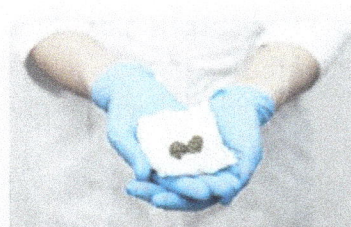

Metabolic Bone Disease

- Osteoporosis and osteomalacia are associated with long-term PN use.
- The exact cause is unknown.
- Contributing factors:

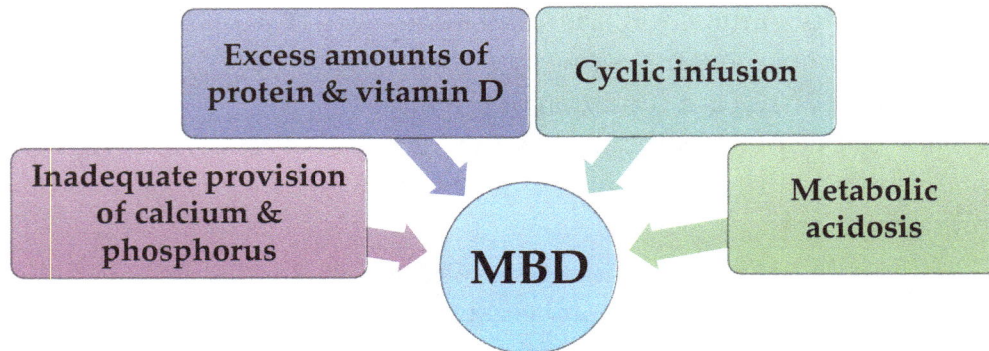

Calcium

- At risk for negative calcium balance due to limited intake and increased urinary calcium loss.
- Higher calcium doses in PN formulas are offset by higher urinary calcium losses.
- Inadequate phosphorus may increase calcium excretion as phosphorus enhances calcium reabsorption by the renal tubules.
- Higher protein doses (2g/kg vs 1g/kg) are associated with increased urinary calcium excretion.
    - Reduce to maintenance dose when possible.
- Chronic metabolic acidosis is associated with hypercalciuria. Correct with acetate.
- Cyclic TPN results in higher urinary losses compared to continuous infusions.

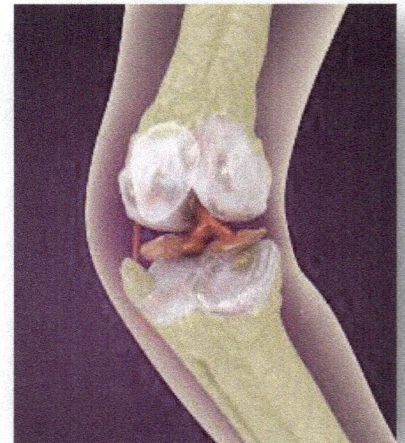

Vitamin D

- Both deficiency and toxicity can result in bone disease.
- PN MVI contains 200 IU ergocalciferol or cholecalciferol.
- Excess doses can suppress PTH (parathyroid hormone) secretion and promote bone resorption.
- The oral route is required to treat deficiency since there are no PN Vitamin D products available.

Aluminum

- Significant aluminum contamination from protein hydrolysates in the past improved with use of crystalline AAs but is still a concern.
- FDA has labeling requirements in large volume parenteral products and required to contain <25mcg Al/liter.

Magnesium

- Hypocalcemia is a prominent manifestation of magnesium deficiency, which results in decreased mobilization of Ca from bone.
  - Chronic severe hypomagnesemia inhibits PTH release resulting in functional hypoparathyroidism.
  - Can also lead to hypophosphatemia due to increased phosphorous excretion.

Copper

- Deficiency impairs bone formation and osteoporosis.

Prevention and Management

- Baseline dual energy x-ray absorptiometry (DEXA) scan recommended for all long term PN patients.

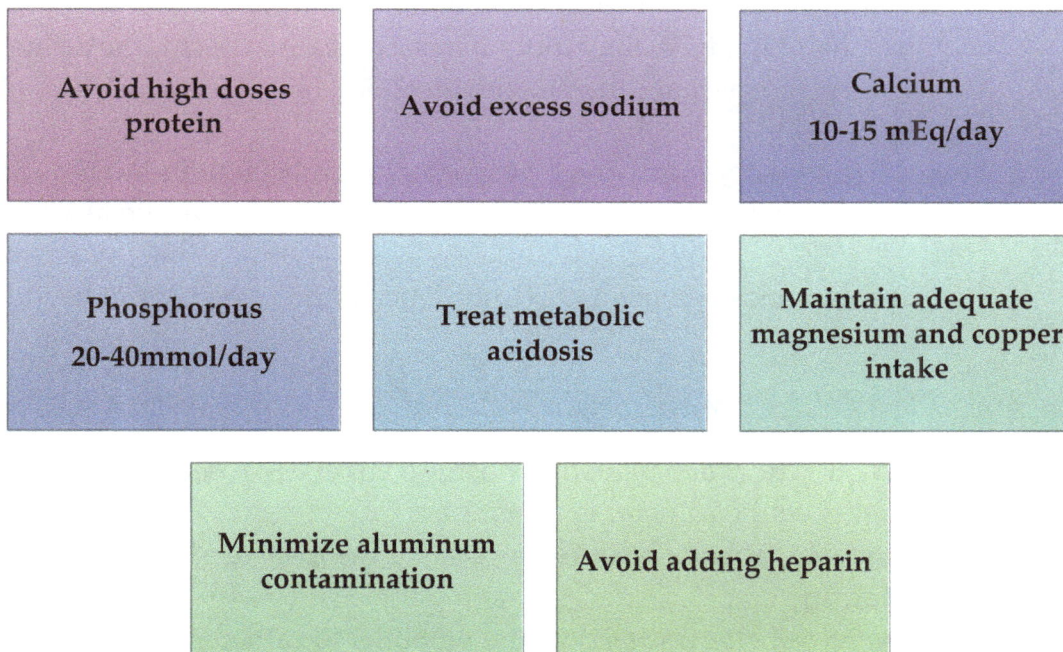

Avoid high doses protein	Avoid excess sodium	Calcium 10-15 mEq/day
Phosphorous 20-40mmol/day	Treat metabolic acidosis	Maintain adequate magnesium and copper intake
Minimize aluminum contamination	Avoid adding heparin	

DEVICE-ASSOCIATED COMPLICATIONS

Catheter-Related Infections

- Hub contamination is the most frequent cause of intraluminal contamination in long term use of VADs
- Gram-positive, coagulase-negative staphylococci is the most prominent pathogen associated with infections from biomedical devices
- Removal of the catheter is recommended for documented fungal infections and *Staph. aureus*
- Coagulase negative staphylococci occur in ~60% of CVC infections in long-term PN patients
- Recurrent gram-negative infections of central lines observed with SBS patients
- Malassezia furfur – superficial fungal infections of the skin and associated structures
  - IVFE presumably provides growth factors for replication of the organism
  - Appropriate treatment: administration of antifungal therapy, discontinuation of IVFE, and removal of the intravascular catheter, especially with non-tunneled catheter infections
- Central Line Bundles and Other Risk Reduction Strategies
  - Includes: hand hygiene, maximum barrier precautions, chlorhexidine skin antisepsis, optimal catheter site selection, daily review of line necessity
  - Use of 70% ethanol-impregnated caps (lock) has been found to reduce the incidence of CRBSIs by >40%, decrease LOS, and lower hospital costs
  - CDC recommends against use of antibiotic ointment on central venous access

Noninfectious Device Complications

- Catheter pinch-off syndrome: related to postural changes caused by catheter compression between the catheter and first rib
  - Changing the patient's position, by raising the ipsilateral arm, relieves the occlusion
  - Can lead to catheter transection and embolus so catheter removal is recommended
  - Pneumothorax as a result of inappropriate placement is a sentinel event

- Thrombophlebitis – swelling or inflammation of vein, often caused by blood clot
  - Presents with swelling and redness at access site
- Device Occlusion – most common noninfectious catheter-related complication
  - Occurs in up to 50% of CVCs (central venous catheters)
  - Presents as inability to flush or pull back on line
- Thrombotic occlusion – primary source of catheter dysfunction and usually due to vessel wall damage, blood flow changes, and systemic alteration in coagulation
  - As catheter size increases, venous blood flow decreases. MAGIC expert panel recommends 1:3 catheter to vein ratio to reduce the risk for catheter-related DVT
  - Risk factors for thrombus formation: catheter tip position, catheter material, type of infusate, length of catheter duration
  - 3 baseline factors with ↑ risk: multiple insertion attempts, ovarian cancer, previous CVC

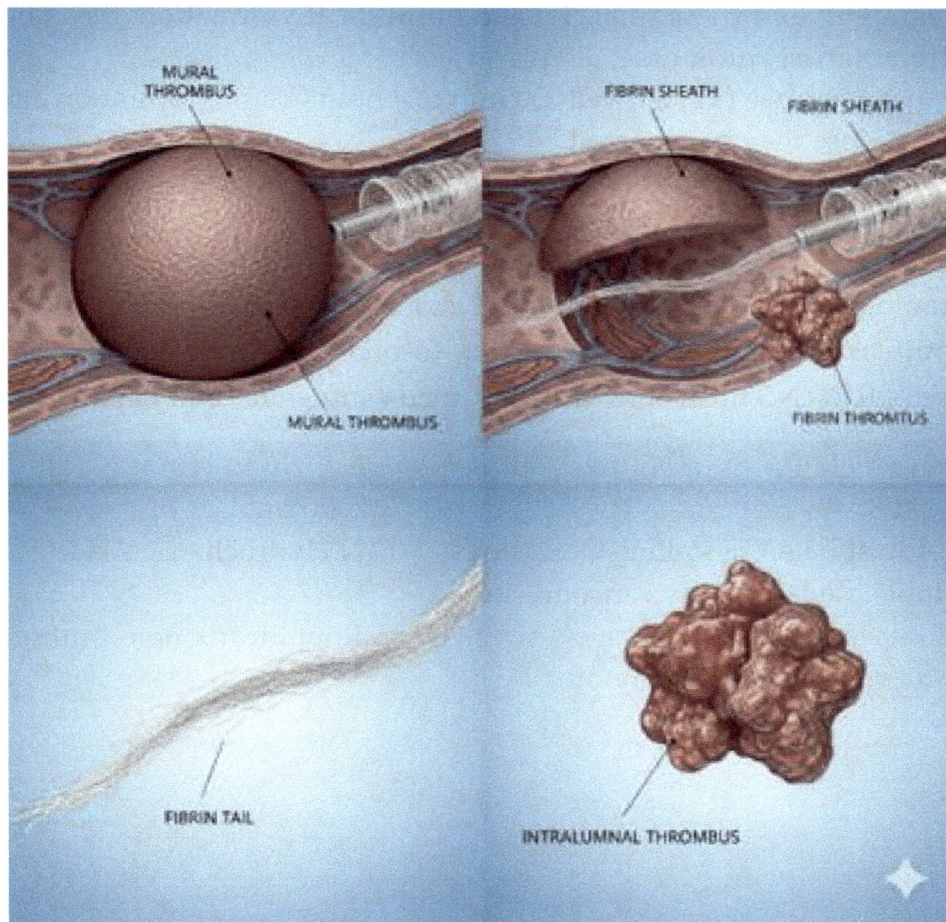

- Mural thrombus
  - Develops when fibrin build up inside the vein causes the vascular access device to adhere to the vessel wall
- Fibrin sheath
  - Layer of fibrin that develops around the outside of a central venous catheter (CVC) secondary to aggregation of fibrin from the presence of a central venous catheter within a vein
- Fibrin tail or flap
  - Fibrin build up on the CVC tip that will allow for infusion through the CVC, but will inhibit withdrawal of blood
- Intraluminal thrombus
  - Clot within the catheter lumen and is caused by inadequate flushing and blood reflux
- SVC thrombosis can result in permanent vascular obstruction/loss of future access
- Treatment for intraluminal clot and fibrin sheath formation: thrombolytics (streptokinase, urokinase, alteplase)
  - Alteplase (TPA) dwells 30 min to 4 hours before aspiration attempted – dose may be repeated
  - If doesn't clear following 2 trials of TPA, replace line

Nonthrombotic Occlusion

- Leading causes of intraluminal occlusions: drug-heparin interactions, PN formulas with inappropriate calcium-to-phosphate ratios, lipid residue
- Use of 0.9% NS flush between all IV meds, infusions, and heparin imperative

Precipitate Causing Occlusion	Treatment
Lipid Residue	70% Ethanol
Calcium-Phosphate/Crystalline Occlusions Acid-Soluble Meds (such as vancomycin)	0.1N Hydrochloric Acid
Base-Soluble Meds (such as tobramycin and phenytoin)	Sodium Bicarbonate 1 mEq/ml

POPULATION-SPECIFIC PN SUPPORT

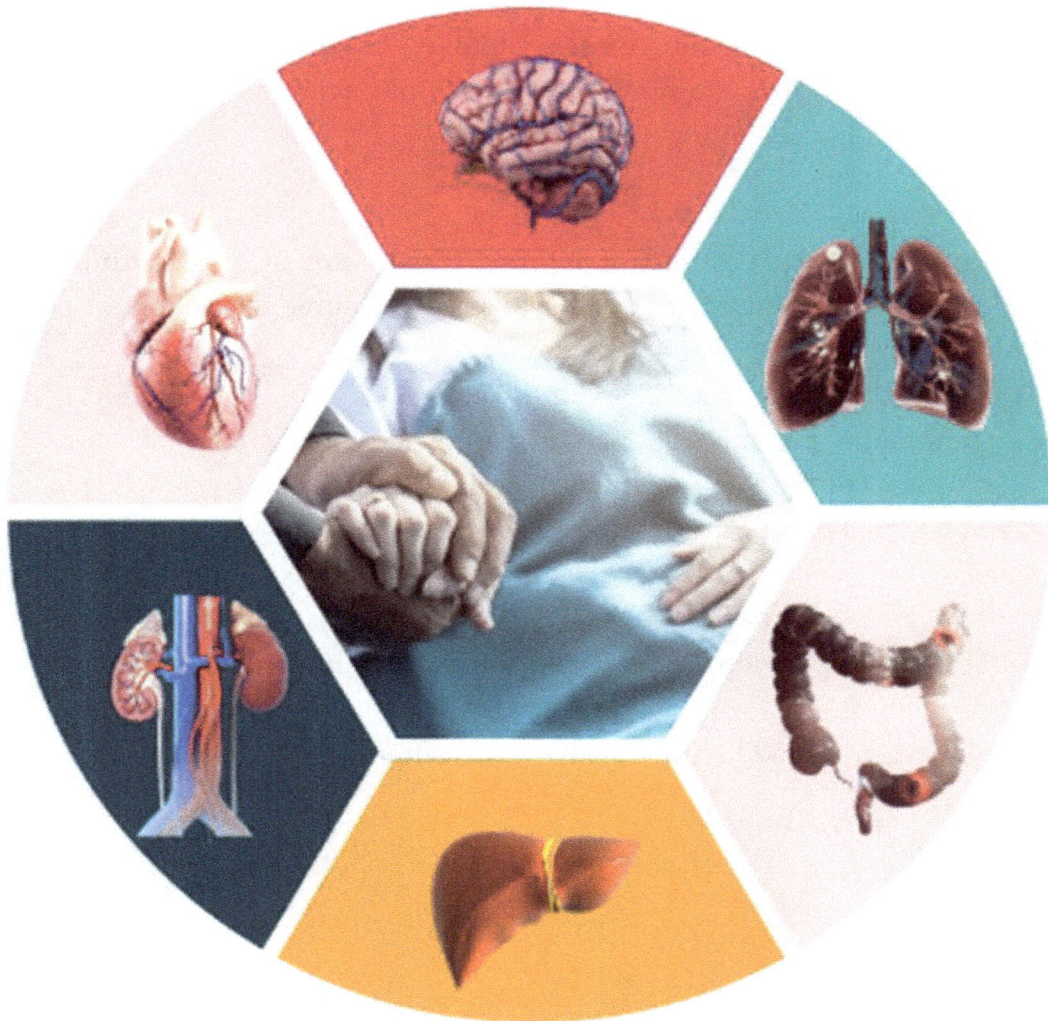

PN in Pregnancy & Hyperemesis

- Indicated in severe cases of hyperemesis gravidarum & IBD complications
- ↑ risk of hyperglycemia – target blood glucose equal to or less than 140 mg/dL
  - May need insulin if DM/GDM present
- TGs increased in pregnancy
  - Normal level = 230 mg/dL
- Presence of ketones in the urine caused by inadequate hydration, hyperglycemia, or inadequate energy intake – helpful in evaluating adequacy
- May need additional vitamin D, vitamin K, folic acid, calcium, magnesium, iron, iodine, and selenium

Renal Impairment & CKD

- May need to start w/ conservative protein & monitor BUN/CRT for tolerance
- High protein load may not be achievable with volume restrictions
- Protein in HD & PD: 1.2-1.4 g/kg/day
- Protein in CRRT: up to 2.0-2.5 g/kg/day
- Use potassium, phosphorus & calcium with caution in CKD
  - Doses of K+, Phos, Mg, Ca2+ should be decreased by 50%
- PD or CRRT dextrose may increase BG levels, so may require additional insulin
- Energy can come from PD solutions: 500-1000kcal
- CRRT can also provide additional calories due to high large amount of replacement fluid
  - Energy from Dialysate: Flow Rate (L/hr) x 24 hrs

Determining Dextrose from PD

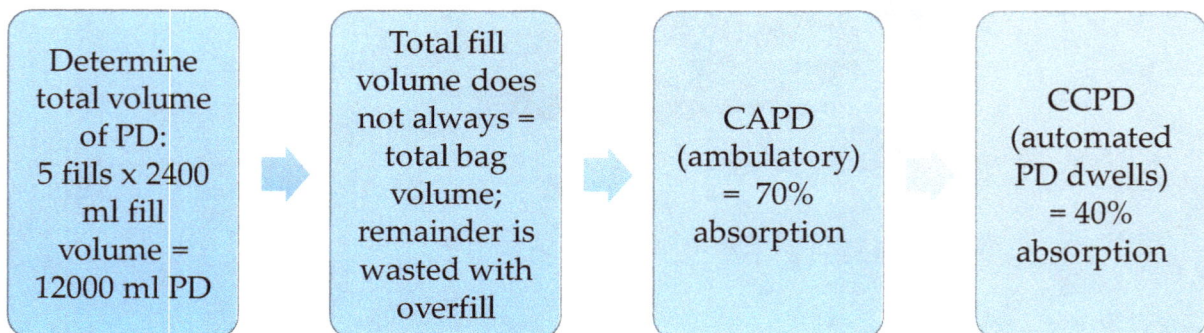

Determine total volume of PD: 5 fills x 2400 ml fill volume = 12000 ml PD	→	Total fill volume does not always = total bag volume; remainder is wasted with overfill	→	CAPD (ambulatory) = 70% absorption	→	CCPD (automated PD dwells) = 40% absorption

Sample Calculation:

- Determine total volume of PD: 5 fills x 2400 mL fill volume = 12000 mL PD

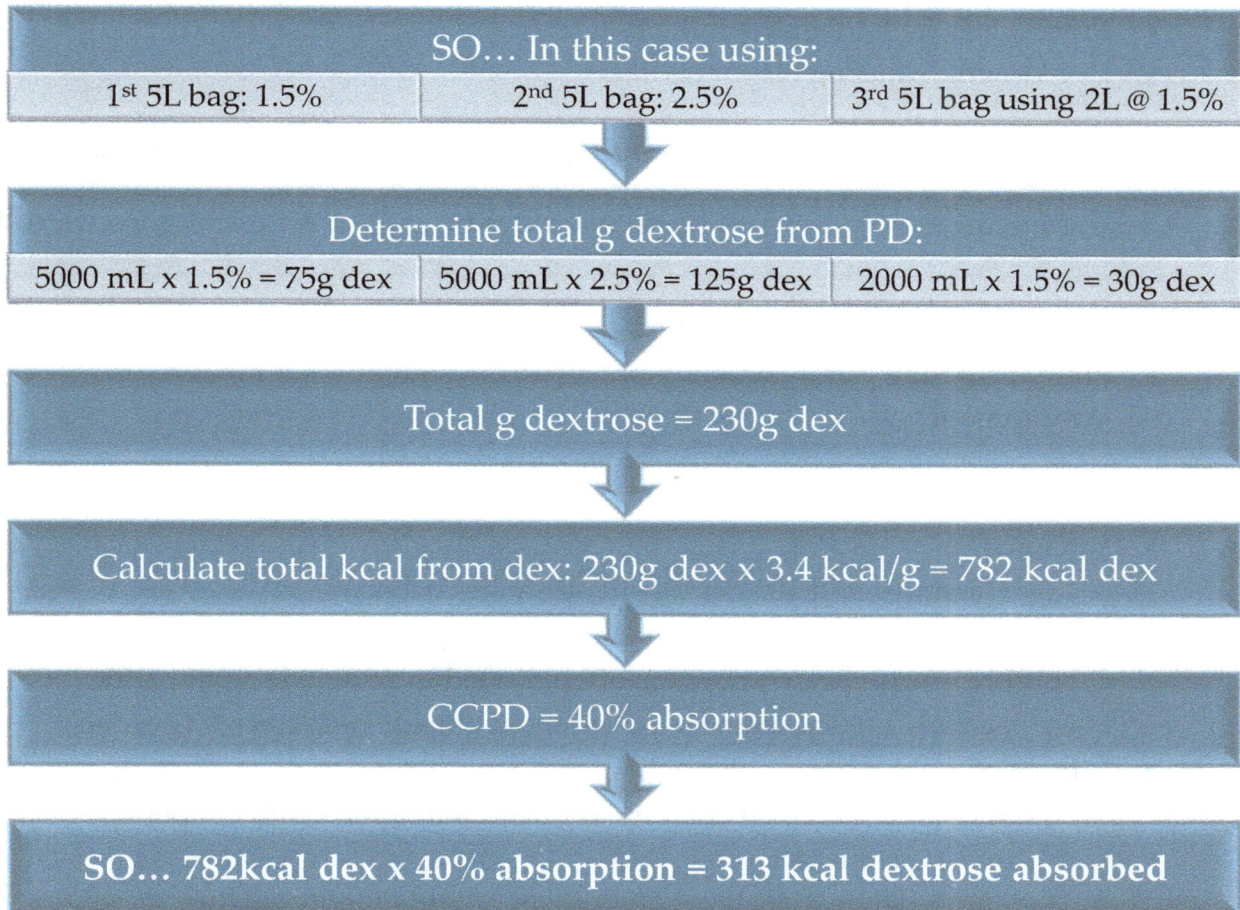

SO… In this case using:		
1st 5L bag: 1.5%	2nd 5L bag: 2.5%	3rd 5L bag using 2L @ 1.5%

⬇

Determine total g dextrose from PD:		
5000 mL x 1.5% = 75g dex	5000 mL x 2.5% = 125g dex	2000 mL x 1.5% = 30g dex

⬇

Total g dextrose = 230g dex

⬇

Calculate total kcal from dex: 230g dex x 3.4 kcal/g = 782 kcal dex

⬇

CCPD = 40% absorption

⬇

SO… 782kcal dex x 40% absorption = 313 kcal dextrose absorbed

Intradialytic PN (IDPN)

- IDPN is parenteral nutrition given during hemodialysis (HD).
- IDPN formulations usually contain protein, dextrose, and lipids, with or without electrolytes, vitamins, and trace elements.
- IDPN typically provides 700 nonprotein kilocalories and 50 to 100 grams of protein in 1 liter per dialysis session (3x/week).
- Standard IDPN contains 100 gm protein, 350 kcal dextrose, and 350 kcal lipids in 1000 ml per HD session.
- Not used much anymore due to inability to meet needs.

Liver Disease

- Energy Needs: 25-30 kcals/day or REE x 1.2-1.4
- Protein Needs: 1-1.5g protein/kg/day
- Dry Weight Adjustments for ascites:

Mild Ascites	Moderate Ascites	Severe Ascites
• 3-5 kg ascitic wt	• 7-9 kg ascitic wt	• 14-15 kg ascitic wt

- Chronic hyponatremia common
- Fluid restriction is not necessary unless serum sodium <125 mmol/L or symptomatic

Micronutrients in Liver Disease

- Vitamins
  - Thiamine: add 100 mg/day in alcoholic cirrhosis
  - Folic Acid: consider additional 1 mg/day in alcoholic cirrhosis
  - Phytonadione (Vitamin K): often needed in acutely coagulopathic patients but should be supplemented outside of PN per MD orders
- Minerals
  - May need to hold if cholestasis due to limitations with copper & manganese clearance
  - Zinc, selenium, & chromium can all be added individually
  - May need supplemental zinc – start with 3 mg/day

Pancreatitis

- **GI or bowel rest and PN no longer have a role in pancreatitis**
- Important to maintain GI integrity with EN as a means to avoid complications from pancreatitis
- Consider glutamine to minimize the effect of being NPO on GI integrity
- Mixed-fuel for PN is preferred with dextrose, protein, and lipids
- Lipids do not exacerbate symptoms of pancreatitis unless the condition is caused by hypertriglyceridemia (usually >1000 mg/Dl) and can be safely started if TG levels < 400 mg/Dl
- If the quantity of lipids in PN is limited to less than 1 g/kg and glucose control is maintained, the risk for hypertriglyceridemia during PN is diminished

ALTERATIONS OF GI TRACT

Inflammatory Bowel Disease

- UC: removal of colon/rectum with end ileostomy or ileal pouch
  - Both have different side effects/issues
- Crohn's – can affect entire GI tract – surgery only option for relief

PN Indications:

- SBS with malabsorption
- (that can't be medically or nutritionally managed)
- Persistent small bowel obstruction
- High-output fistulas
- Enteric fistulas originating in a location that do not allow EN distal to the fistula
- Provide perioperative support to severely malnourished patients for 1-2 weeks prior to surgery

Micronutrient Considerations

- Ileal resections increase risk of B12 deficiency
- Zinc deficiency from high output fistulas or frequent diarrhea
  - Monitor copper stores with zinc supplementation

Perioperative Malnutrition

- Stress of surgical procedures produces an abundance of proinflammatory cytokines, which increase metabolic rate and cause catabolism, resulting in a depletion of lean body mass and aberrations in glycemic control
- Patients at the highest risk of diverse postsurgical outcomes are those with low visceral protein stores (specifically albumin) at baseline
- Early NS in pre- and postop phases associated with better patient outcomes
- Maximal benefit is derived in severely malnourished patients who receive PN for more than 7-10 days

Supplemental PN (SPN)

ASPEN/SCCM (2016): Indicated for cumulative caloric deficit w/ EN ≤60% needs over ≥ 10 days	→	Many newer studies suggest role for early SPN around day 3-4 when EN indaquate

Early SPN significantly increased energy and protein provision and decreased infectious complications, with no statistically significant difference in noninfectious complications, total adverse events, vent duration, ICU admit, or hospital length of stay.

Ostomies

- End ostomy completely diverts GI contents at abdominal wall level, while loop ostomy maintains partial continuity

Indications for ileostomy	Indications for colostomy
• Emergent subtotal colectomy • Anastomotic protection • Distal small bowel injuries	o Colon injuries in high-risk patients o Obstruction from intra-abdominal malignancy

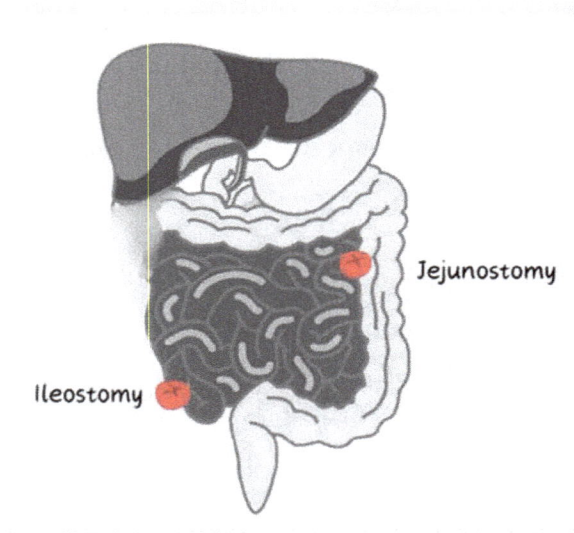

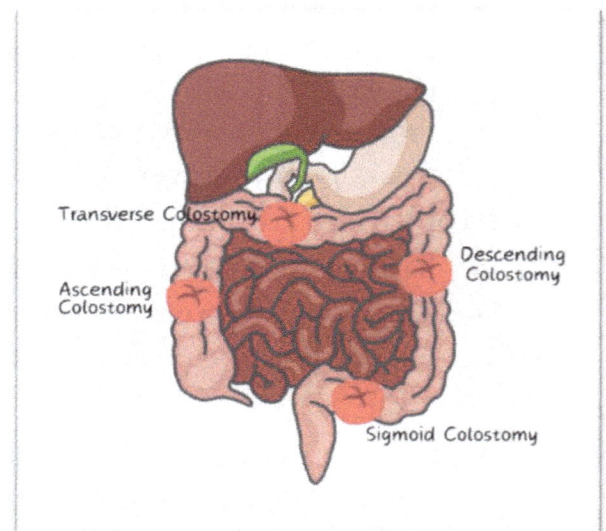

Typical Ostomy Output

Colostomy	200 – 600 mL/day
Ileostomy	>1200 initially post-op, decreasing to average 750 mL/day
Jejunostomy	Can be up to 6 L/day initially

- Normal stool output in intact GI tract = < 200 mL/day
- Ostomies can lead to fluid/electrolyte imbalances
    - High ostomy output
        - Ileostomy > 1 L/24 hrs
        - Colostomy > 600 mL/24 hrs
    - Manage with fiber supplementation and antimotility agents

Enterocutaneous Fistulas

- Most ECFs (75% to 80%) result from surgical complications (i.e., unrecognized enterotomy, anastomotic leaks), while some develop spontaneously due to ongoing inflammation (i.e., Crohn's disease)
- Metabolic complications of ECFs:
    - Fluid and electrolyte imbalance
    - D-lactic acidosis
    - Micronutrient deficiencies
    - Osteoporosis and osteomalacia
- ECF management

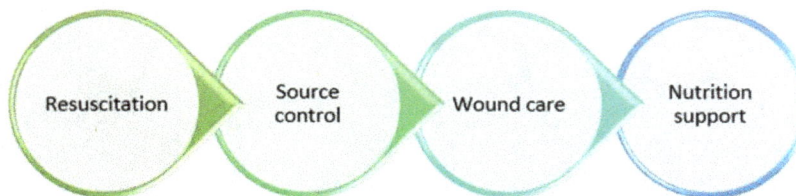

Resuscitation → Source control → Wound care → Nutrition support

    - NPO + PN significantly reduced ECF-associated mortality
    - Supplementation of trace minerals, zinc, copper, and vitamins
- Low-output ECFs often close within 4 weeksEnteral feeding through a tube directly into the fistula can be used in patients with proximal ECFs or low output fistulas (<500 ml)
- If feeding via the GI tract is initiated, it should be controlled using antimotility agents and electrolyte monitoring

Chylothorax, Chylous Ascites, & Chyle Leaks

Chylothorax	Chylous ascites
• Presence of chyle within the pleural space	• Presence of chyle within the peritoneal cavity

- Conservative management: high-protein, very-low-fat, and MCT supplemented diet recommended
- PN may be used if EN is not tolerated, but care should be taken to prevent essential fatty acid deficiency when restricting long-chain fatty acids for over two weeks
- Long-term PN administration can significantly reduce chyle flow rates from postprandial levels to fasting rate

SHORT BOWEL SYNDROME (SBS)

- Defined as < 200 cm functional small bowel
- Length of residual small bowel determines the severity of SBS, other factors strongly influence net intestinal absorption
- Healthy small bowel absorbs a daily average of 6-8 liters of fluid
- Clinically significant symptoms of SBS don't appear until ¾ of the original small bowel has been resected

Anatomical Variants of SBS

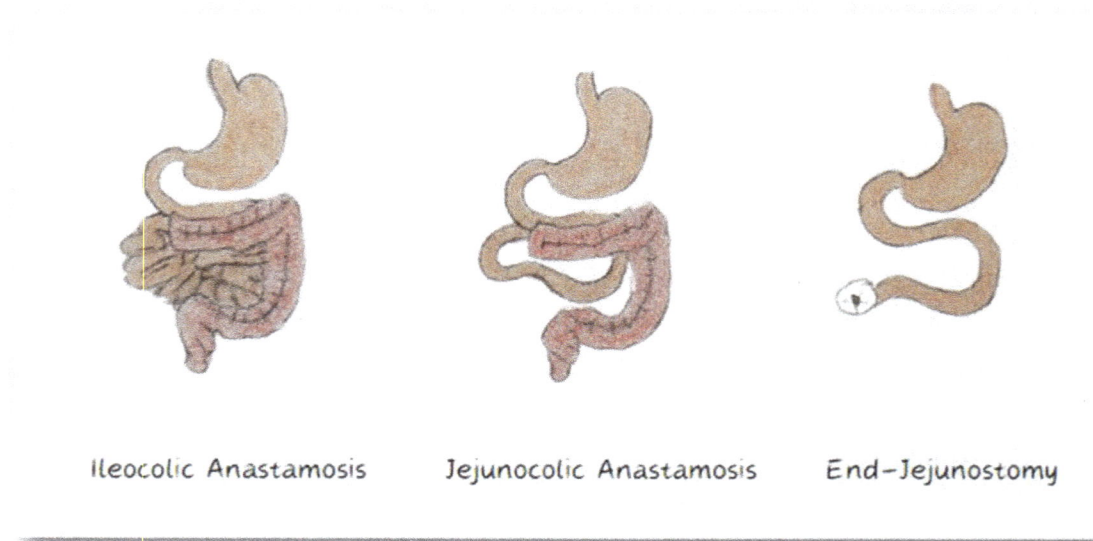

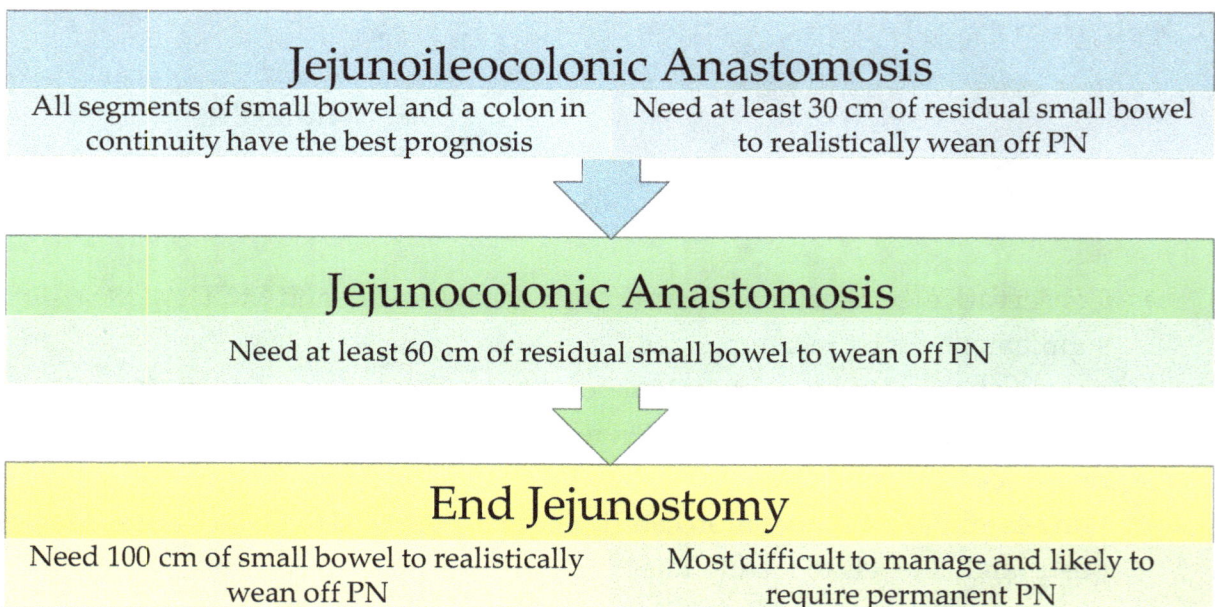

| Ileocolic Anastamosis | Jejunocolic Anastamosis | End-Jejunostomy |

Jejunoileocolonic Anastomosis

All segments of small bowel and a colon in continuity have the best prognosis

Need at least 30 cm of residual small bowel to realistically wean off PN

Jejunocolonic Anastomosis

Need at least 60 cm of residual small bowel to wean off PN

End Jejunostomy

Need 100 cm of small bowel to realistically wean off PN

Most difficult to manage and likely to require permanent PN

Altered Absorption

- **Most stable patients with SBS absorb about half to a third of the energy that healthy individuals absorb**
- Intestinal adaptation occurs over 1-2 years and is associated with progressive improvement in nutrient and fluid absorption
- The ileum's active transport of sodium chloride allows for significant fluid reabsorption and the ability to concentrate the contents of the ileum
  - Sodium concentration in the jejunostomy fluid is about 90-140 mEq/L
- Terminal ileum is the main site of carrier mediated absorption of B12 and enterohepatic recirculation of bile
  - When less than 100 cm of terminal ileum is resected, upregulated hepatic synthesis of bile can compensate for losses of unrecycled bile
  - When more than 100 cm of the terminal ileum is resected, the amount of unrecycled bile loss exceeds the maximum rate of hepatic synthesis of bile, leading to bile insufficiency, fat malabsorption and steatorrhea
- Large-volume diarrhea leads to significant water loss and electrolyte wasting
  - Hydration strategies can be tailored for a goal urine output of more than 1 L/d and a urinary sodium concentration greater than 20 mEq/L
- Fat-soluble vitamin and EFA deficiencies are also commonly encountered
- Supplemental zinc and, occasionally, selenium may be required in the presence of excessive stool losses

PN Support in SBS

- Anatomy, length, and integrity of residual small bowel are strong predictors of long-term need for PN
- A prognostic biomarker of intestinal function is citrulline, a nonessential amino acid found to correlate with eventual independence from PN when serum levels are greater than 15-20 mcmol/L
- In the presence of a high ostomy output, fluid, potassium, magnesium, and zinc losses can increase and would need vigilant monitoring and repletion
- When calculating PN volume and content, clinicians should monitor changes in patient's weight, energy levels, lab test data, stool or ostomy output, urine output, and complaints of thirst
- SBS patients on PN remain at risk for micronutrient deficiencies; therefore, micronutrient levels require periodic monitoring, and supplementation should be used in addition to PN

Parenteral Hydration

- Patients may attain gut autonomy for macronutrients but still require parenteral fluid supplementation despite optimization of diet and ORS supplementation
- The IVF is commonly provided as a liter of normal saline infused over a couple of hours once daily as needed
- The contents of the fluid may include only sodium chloride or dextrose; other electrolytes, vitamins, and bicarbonate may occasionally be added

Oral Rehydration Solutions (ORS)

- Ostomy output should be controlled before ORS use
- It's very important to counsel patients that commercial sports drinks are not acceptable substitutes for oral rehydration solutions as they contain less sodium and more sugar than patients need for best absorption
- Recipes from *A Patient's Guide to Managing a Short Bowel* (Carol Rees Parrish MS, RD)

Regular Sports Drink	Low-Calorie Sports Drink	WHO ORS
• 1.5 cups sports drink • 2.5 cups water • 1/2 tsp salt • Equates to 1 L	• 1 qt ready-to-drink low-calorie sports drink • 1/4-1/2 tsp salt • Equates to 1 L	• 4.25 cups water • 1/2 tsp salt • 2 tbsp sugar • Equates to 1 L

Intestinal Rehabilitation

- Strategies include:
  - Reduction of meal sizes with an increased number of meals
  - Restriction of fluid intake during meals
  - Reduced consumption of hypertonic fluids
  - Use of ORS for hydration
  - Titration of antidiarrheals
  - Consideration of intestinal trophic agents
- Before PN is reduced, patients should also meet certain criteria:
  - Adequate hydration (UOP greater than 1 L/day)
  - Ability to consistently consume at least 80% of daily energy goals
  - Weight stability or gains
  - Stability of serum electrolyte levels
  - Oral fluid intake minus stool and urine output greater than 500 mL/d

SUMMARY OF GI TRACT ALTERATIONS

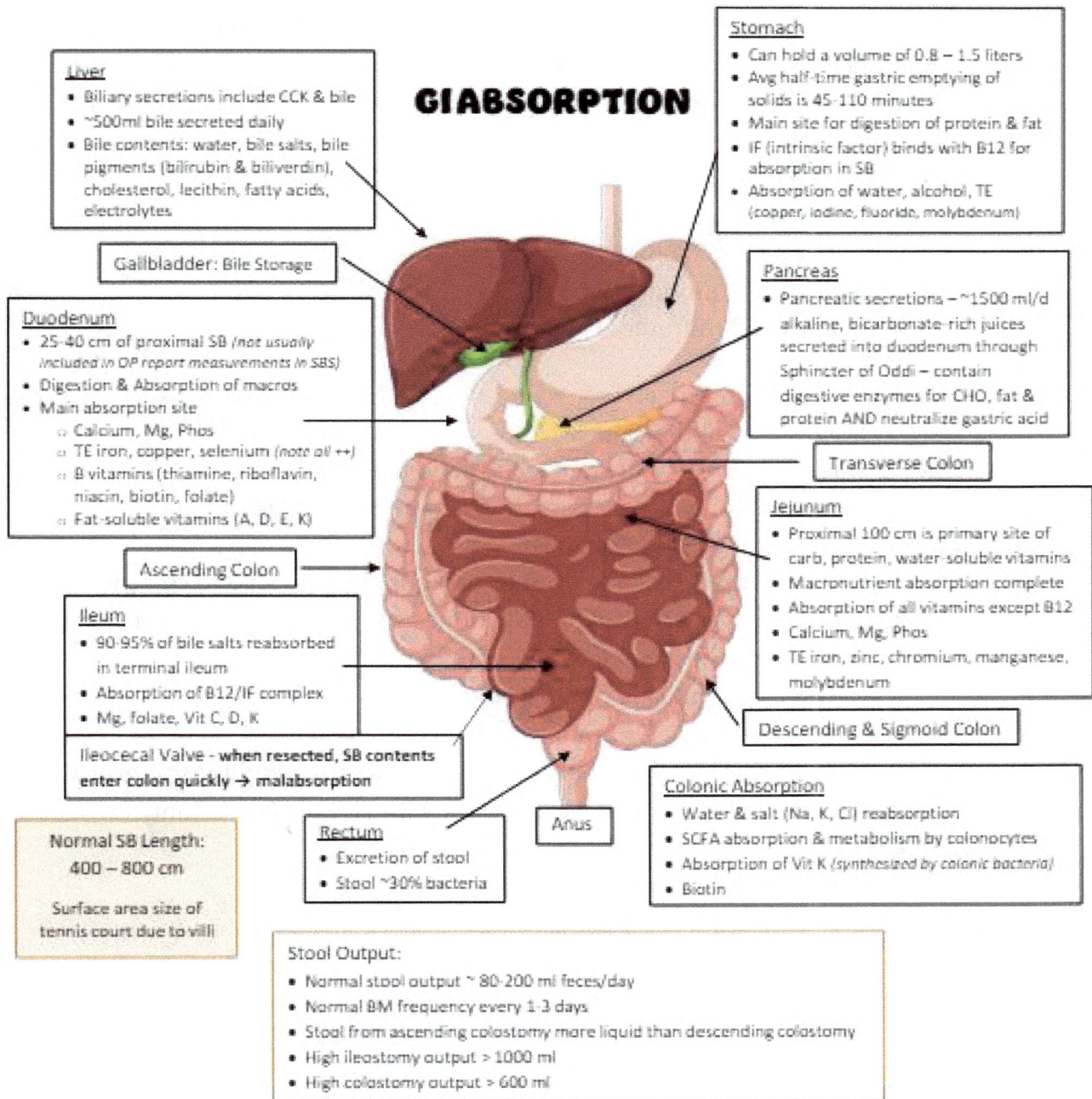

GI ABSORPTION

Liver
- Biliary secretions include CCK & bile
- ~500ml bile secreted daily
- Bile contents: water, bile salts, bile pigments (bilirubin & biliverdin), cholesterol, lecithin, fatty acids, electrolytes

Gallbladder: Bile Storage

Duodenum
- 25-40 cm of proximal SB (not usually included in OP report measurements in SBS)
- Digestion & Absorption of macros
- Main absorption site
  - Calcium, Mg, Phos
  - TE iron, copper, selenium (note all ++)
  - B vitamins (thiamine, riboflavin, niacin, biotin, folate)
  - Fat-soluble vitamins (A, D, E, K)

Ascending Colon

Ileum
- 90-95% of bile salts reabsorbed in terminal ileum
- Absorption of B12/IF complex
- Mg, folate, Vit C, D, K

Ileocecal Valve - when resected, SB contents **enter colon quickly → malabsorption**

Normal SB Length:
400 – 800 cm

Surface area size of tennis court due to villi

Rectum
- Excretion of stool
- Stool ~30% bacteria

Anus

Stomach
- Can hold a volume of 0.8 – 1.5 liters
- Avg half-time gastric emptying of solids is 45-110 minutes
- Main site for digestion of protein & fat
- IF (intrinsic factor) binds with B12 for absorption in SB
- Absorption of water, alcohol, TE (copper, iodine, fluoride, molybdenum)

Pancreas
- Pancreatic secretions – ~1500 ml/d alkaline, bicarbonate-rich juices secreted into duodenum through Sphincter of Oddi – contain digestive enzymes for CHO, fat & protein AND neutralize gastric acid

Transverse Colon

Jejunum
- Proximal 100 cm is primary site of carb, protein, water-soluble vitamins
- Macronutrient absorption complete
- Absorption of all vitamins except B12
- Calcium, Mg, Phos
- TE iron, zinc, chromium, manganese, molybdenum

Descending & Sigmoid Colon

Colonic Absorption
- Water & salt (Na, K, Cl) reabsorption
- SCFA absorption & metabolism by colonocytes
- Absorption of Vit K (synthesized by colonic bacteria)
- Biotin

Stool Output:
- Normal stool output ~ 80-200 ml feces/day
- Normal BM frequency every 1-3 days
- Stool from ascending colostomy more liquid than descending colostomy
- High ileostomy output > 1000 ml
- High colostomy output > 600 ml

BARIATRIC SURGERY

Types of Bariatric Surgery Procedures

- Roux-en-Y Gastric Bypass (RYGB): divides the stomach into a remnant (nonfunctional) stomach and a small gastric pouch that remains in continuity; the duodenum is bypassed to decrease absorption and the gastric pouch is connected into the small bowel approximately 3-4 feet downstream, resulting in a bowel connection resembling the shape of the letter Y
    - Restrictive & malabsorptive
- Complications of RYGB:
    - Nausea & vomiting
    - Dumping Syndrome
    - Ulcers
    - Hypoglycemia
    - Micronutrient deficiencies
- Sleeve Gastrectomy: 80% of stomach is removed
    - Restrictive only; fewer micronutrient deficiencies compared to procedures involving bypass
    - Gastric content leakage from transection line can lead to complications
- Biliopancreatic Diversion (BPD): often done as BPD-DS with duodenal switch – combination of sleeve gastrectomy with bypass of duodenum
    - Restrictive & malabsorptive (more so than RYGB)
    - Also affects bowel hormones to increase satiety
    - Greater risk of nutritional deficiencies but best weight loss efficacy
- Single Anastomosis Duodeno-Ileal Bypass with Sleeve Gastrectomy (SADI-S): similar to BPD-DS but only 1 intestinal anastomosis
    - Often used as 2nd stage surgery following sleeve
    - Newer procedure so limited data

TYPES OF BARIATRIC SURGERY

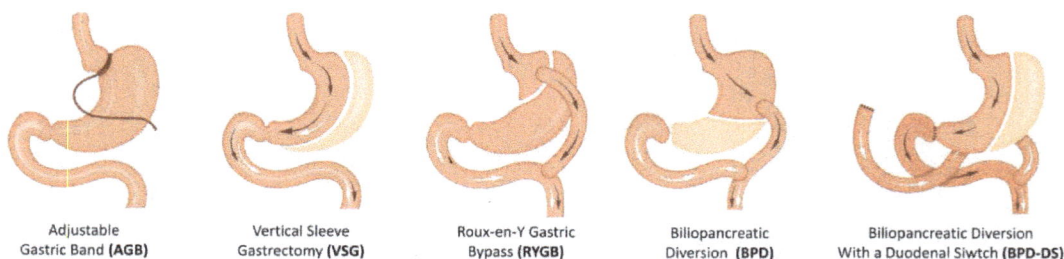

| Adjustable Gastric Band (AGB) | Vertical Sleeve Gastrectomy (VSG) | Roux-en-Y Gastric Bypass (RYGB) | Biliopancreatic Diversion (BPD) | Biliopancreatic Diversion With a Duodenal Siwtch (BPD-DS) |

PN in Bariatric Malnutrition & Failure to Thrive

- TPN is rarely needed after bariatric surgery
- When used, it is most commonly initiated because of either infectious complication (leak, perforation, abscess) or noninfectious failure to thrive
- Noninfectious Failure to Thrive
    - Chronic ulcer disease
    - Recurrent obstruction
    - Anastomotic strictures
    - Incisional hernias
    - Other food intolerance
- Patients requiring TPN for infectious indications including leak, perforation, and abscess tend to have more severe malnutrition (despite a higher BMI) and more prolonged hospital stays than those with noninfectious failure to thrive
- Follow refeeding guidelines if malnutrition present
- Include daily thiamine 100 mg/day in TPN

Micronutrient Deficiencies Post Bariatric Surgery

- Fat Soluble Vitamins A, D, E, K
- Thiamine, Vitamin B6, Vitamin B12 *(loss of intrinsic factor)*
- Minerals: Iron & Zinc
- Malabsorption and micronutrient deficiencies are more common after gastric bypass and duodenal switch

Needs Assessment in the Obese Patient

- ESPEN: 20-25 kcal/kg & > 1.0 g protein/kg based on adjusted BW in acute care
    - Increase protein to >1.3 g/kg/d critical care
    - 25 kcal/kg Adj BW appropriate for most patients unless weight loss indicated

Critical Illness

- Gut failure is common because of preferential blood supply to vital organs
- Mesenteric ischemia resulting from hemodynamic compromise and the use of vasopressors is a potential problem
- PN reserved for those cases when EN cannot be initiated for >7 days
- PN should only be initiated in patients who are hemodynamically stable and who can tolerate the fluid volume and protein, CHO and ILE doses necessary to provide adequate nutrient substrate

ASPEN/SCCM Critical Care Guidelines for PN

- In low risk patients (NRS 2002 ≤ 3 or NUTRIC score ≤ 5), exclusive PN should be withheld in the first 7 days following ICU admission when po/EN is contraindicated
- When EN is not feasible in high-risk (NRS or NUTRIC ≥ 5) or severely malnourished patients, consider initiating exclusive PN as soon as possible following ICU admission
- Consider use of supplemental PN after 7-10 days if patient unable to meet >60% energy and protein needs via enteral route alone
- Protocols and nutrition support teams should be utilized to incorporate strategies to maximize efficiency and minimize PN-associated risks
- In high-risk or severely malnourished patients receiving PN, consider hypocaloric dosing (≤ 20 kcal/kg/d or 80% EER) with adequate protein (≥1.2 g/kg/d) initially over first week of ICU hospitalization

> **When in this acute phase of sepsis, ASPEN guidelines suggest not using exclusive PN or supplemental PN in conjunction with EN, regardless of the patient's degree of nutrition risk**

PN in the COVID Patient

- Indications for PN:
    - Threshold for switching to PN lower in COVID disease where increased concern for ischemic bowel & prolonged ICU stay expected
    - Early PN in moderately to severely malnourished patients and those identified as high risk with NUTRIC score ≥ 5 or NRS score ≥ 5 if early gastric EN not feasible
    - COVID with GI involvement (nausea, vomiting, diarrhea, GI bleeding) – indicates greater disease severity
    - Previously healthy individuals can delay PN 5-7 days, while monitored every 3-4 days
- Withhold soybean lipids or use alternative mixed lipid emulsions (SMOF) in 1st week of ICU stay
- Monitor serum triglycerides within 24 hours of PN initiation if also receiving Propofol

Cancer

- Routine PN use in patients receiving chemotherapy or radiation is associated with increased infectious complications and no improvement in clinical response, survival, or toxicity to chemotherapy

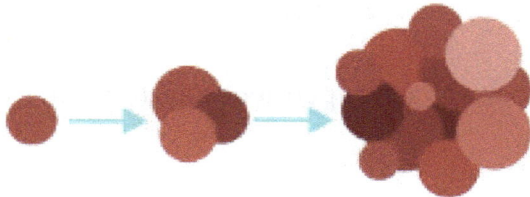

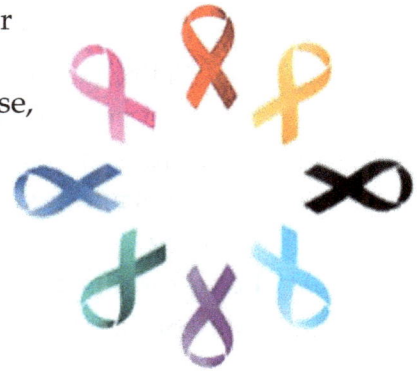

- EN is preferred in patients undergoing a hematopoietic cell transplant because glycemic control is better
- Home PN:
  - Might be needed for short bowel syndrome, high output GI or pancreatic fistulas, bowel obstructions, or prolonged radiation enteritis
  - ASPEN guidelines suggest that palliative use of PN in terminally ill cancer patients is rarely indicated
  - Patient must need PN for at least 3 months, therefore patients with life expectancy of 40-60 days would not qualify
  - Patients on aggressive treatments with good performance status, inoperable bowel obstruction, or patients with minimal symptoms of the disease are the best candidates for short term PN

HOME PN SUPPORT

- *Ideally should* be cycled prior to discharge home (usually 12-14 hrs nocturnally)
  - TPN macros should be at goal & tolerated before cycling
- BG must be maintained < 180 mg/dL
- Potassium must not exceed 10 mEq/L per hour
- Vitamins and insulin provided separately & must be added to TPN prior to hanging
- Long-term goals are promoting patient's independence and preventing rehospitalization.

Medicare Guidelines:

- Medicare requires documentation that the patient's GI tract is nonfunctional, and the condition is permanent – at least 90 days of therapy is needed

HOME PN MEDICARE GUIDELINES	
Dextrose	$\geqq$ 10%
Protein	0.8-1.5 g/kg/day
Lipids	$\geqq$ 2%
Total kcal	20-35 kcal/kg/day

Eligibility & documentation of medical necessity for HPN

- **Permanent dysfunction of the alimentary tract**
  - Permanent defined > 3 months
- Documented evidence of inability to tolerate EN (malabsorption, obstruction)
- Swallowing disorders, psychological disorders, anorexia, dyspnea of severe pulmonary or cardiac disease, medication side effects, or renal failure NOT routinely covered
- PN prescription must meet specified calorie and protein guidelines
- Reimbursement for lipids limited by Medicare guidelines
- Medicare covers rental of infusion pumps and cost of supplies for those who meet PN eligibility criteria
- Does not generally pay for nursing care for administration of feedings, but it offers limited coverage for teaching the patient/family how to administer infusions

Determining safety of home environment for HNS

- Access to home care agencies
- Clean environment with reliable utilities
  - Includes refrigeration & access to telephone
- Patient able to move safely around the house
- Patient or caregiver willing & able to learn home infusion procedures & operation of equipment
- Patient or caregiver able to recognize problems & contact home healthcare provider or emergency services
- Laboratory monitoring available
- No history of substance use disorder

Patient/Caregiver education for home nutrition support should include formula schedule, preparation and administration, formula storage, access safety & sanitation

Home PN Administration

- Long-term PN requires central venous access device – Peripheral & midlines should NOT be used for HPN due to easy dislodgement, need for routine changes, & inability to handle high-osmolarity solutions
  - Peripherally inserted central catheter (PICC) should only be used for short-term therapy (< 3 months) due to risks of displacement, loss of patency, & increased thrombosis risk with longer term use
  - Subclavian or internal jugular catheters are either tunneled or implanted – enter the vein & tunneled subcutaneously to exit lower on chest wall
    - Tunneled catheters – Hickman, Broviac, PowerLine, Hohn, Groshong - tunneled to decrease risks of infection & accidental removal
    - Implanted device (port) is disk with self-sealing silicone septum & rigid titanium or plastic base
- PN cycle should include tapered rate at the end of infusion to minimize risk of hypoglycemia = 1 hour at the beginning of infusion & 1-2 hours at the end of the infusion
  - Careful glucose monitoring needed while infusion rate is increased = Glucose utilization rate is between 4 and 7 mg/kg/min (generally accepted rate of glucose infusion being 5 mg/kg/min)

- Home insulin administration = Sliding scale or addition of regular insulin to PN solution
    - Patients & caregivers must receive adequate education on dose, proper syringe, needle size, & technique for adding insulin to the PN bag
    - May have basal insulin requirements met by insulin in PN solution while breakthrough elevations are covered by cutaneous injections
- Laboratory Monitoring for HPN
    - Trace elements, vitamins, and the phospholipid fatty acid profile (triene: tetraene ratio) should be checked every 3-12 months, with more frequent monitoring for patients with known deficiencies or toxicities, or when national shortages of IV trace elements, vitamins, or lipids occur
    - Triene: tetraene ratio is gold standard for EFAD assessment – should be evaluated for patients receiving lipid-free, lipid-minimized HPN, or lipids with decreased levels of omega-6 fatty acids
- Monitoring - Office visits should be scheduled for 1 month after start of therapy with the physician & nutrition support clinician & then every 3 to 6 months while nutrition support continues

REFERENCES

1. Chan L-N, et al (Eds.). *The ASPEN Adult Nutrition Support Core Curriculum, 4th Edition.* ASPEN 2025.

2. Mueller CM, et al (Eds). *The ASPEN Adult Nutrition Support Core Curriculum, 3rd Edition.* ASPEN 2017.

3. Compher C, Bingham AL, McCall M, et al. Guidelines for the Provision and Assessment of Nutrition Support Therapy in the Adult Critically Ill Patient: the American Society for Parenteral and Enteral Nutrition. JPEN. 2022; 1-30. https://doi.org/10.1002/jpen.2267

4. McClave, SA et al. Guidelines for the Provision and Assessment of Nutrition Support Therapy in the Adult Critically Ill Patient: Society of Critical Care Medicine (SCCM) and American Society for Parenteral and Enteral Nutrition (A.S.P.E.N.). JPEN. 2016: 40 (2): 159-211. http://sccmmedia.sccm.org/documents/LearnICU/Guidelines/Nutrition-SCCM-ASPEN.pdf

5. Ayers, P., Adams, S., Boullata, J., Gervasio, J., Holcombe, B., Kraft, M.D., Marshall, N., Neal, A., Sacks, G., Seres, D.S., Worthington, P. and (2014), A.S.P.E.N. Parenteral Nutrition Safety Consensus Recommendations. Journal of Parenteral and Enteral Nutrition, 38: 296-333. https://doi.org/10.1177/0148607113511992

6. Bruno J, et al. A.S.P.E.N. Fluids, Electrolytes, and Acid-Base Disorders Handbook. Silver Springs: American Society for Parenteral and Enteral Nutrition, 2020.

7. Ayers P, et al. A.S.P.E.N. Parenteral Nutrition Handbook, 3rd Edition. Silver Springs: American Society for Parenteral and Enteral Nutrition, 2020.

8. White JV, Guenter P, et al. Consensus Statement: Academy of Nutrition and Dietetics and American Society for Parenteral and Enteral Nutrition: Characteristics Recommended for the Identification and Documentation of Adult Malnutrition (Under-nutrition). JPEN J Parent Ent Nutr. 2012; 36:275-283.

9. da Silva, J.S.V. et al. ASPEN Consensus Recommendations for Refeeding Syndrome. *Nutrition in Clinical Practice,* 2020; 35: 178-195. https://doi.org/10.1002/ncp.10474.

10. Ponzo, V., Pellegrini, M., Cioffi, I. et al. The Refeeding Syndrome: a neglected but potentially serious condition for inpatients. A narrative review. Intern Emerg Med, 16, 49–60 (2021). https://doi.org/10.1007/s11739-020-02525-7.

11. Naik NM, Li J, Seres D, Freedberg DE. Assessment of refeeding syndrome definitions and 30-day mortality in critically ill adults: A comparison study. JPEN J Parenter Enteral Nutr. 2023; 47: 993-1002. https://doi.org/10.1002/jpen.2560.

12. Parrish, CR (2015). *A Patient's Guide to Managing a Short Bowel, 3rd Edition.*

13. Mechanik JI, et al. Clinical practice guidelines for the perioperative nutrition, metabolic, and nonsurgical support of patients undergoing bariatric procedures – 2019 update: cosponsored by American Association of Clinical Endocrinologists/American College of Endocrinology, The Obesity Society, American Society for Metabolic & Bariatric Surgery, Obesity Medicine Association, and American Society of Anesthesiologists. Surgery for Obesity and Related Diseases, 16 (2020) 175–247.

14. Osland E, et al. Micronutrient management following bariatric surgery: the role of the dietitian in the postoperative period. Ann Transl Med 2020;8(Suppl 1): S9. doi: 10.21037/atm.2019.06.04

APPENDICES

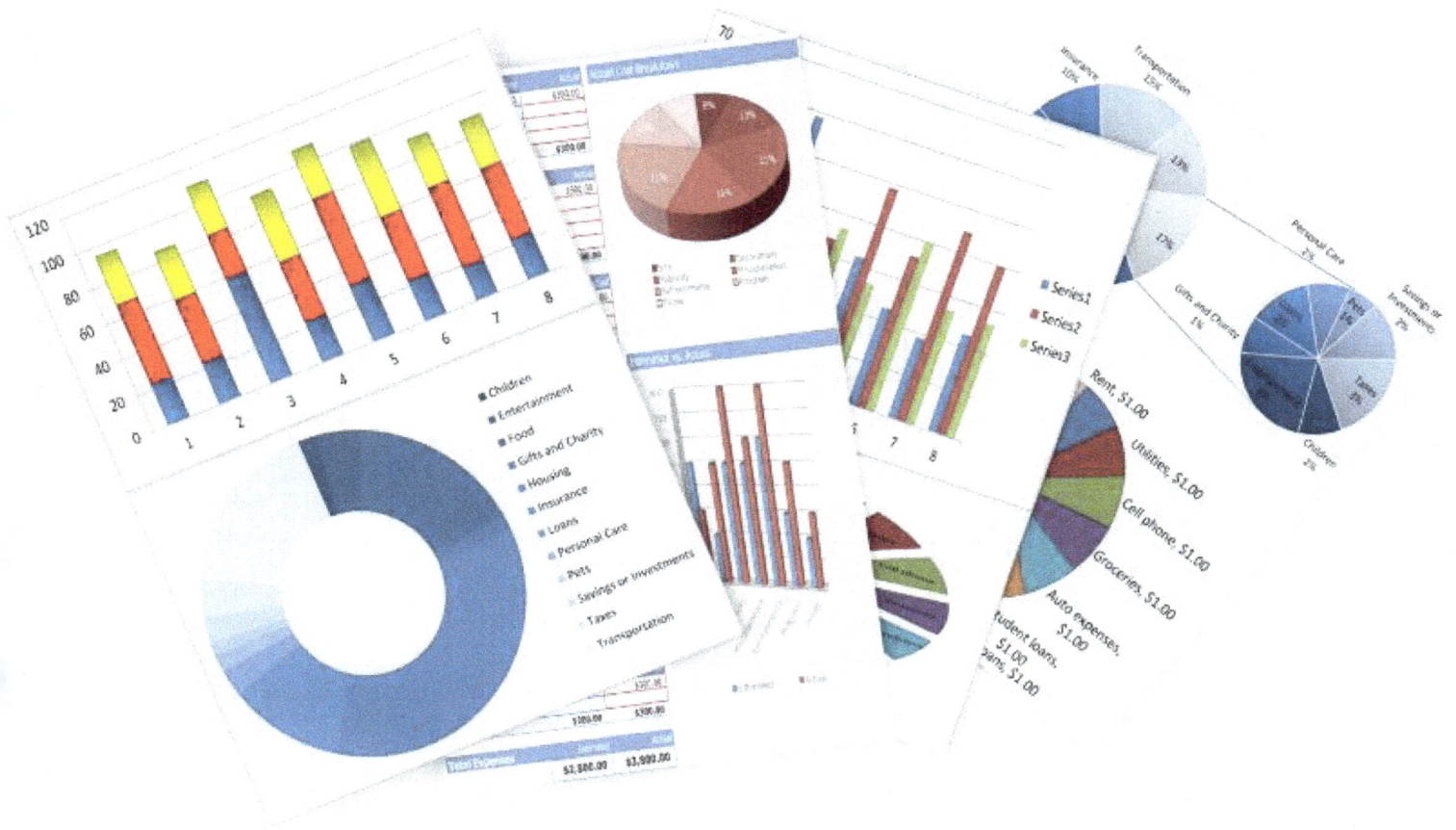

PN WORKSHEET

Patient Name/Room: _____

MRN: _____ DOB: _____ PMH: _____

Admit Wt: _____ Ht: _____ BMI: _____ Dosing Weight: _____

Indication for PN: _____

RD Goal Macros AA: (/kg) Dextrose: _____ Lipids: _____ IL or SMOF KCAL: _____ /kg: _____

Labs & Daily Assessment

Date										
Wt										
Na (136-144)										
K (3.6-5.1)										
Cl (101-111)										
CO2 (22-29)										
Gluc (74-118)										
BUN (8-20)										
CRT (0.4-1.0)										
Ca (8.9-10.3)										
Corrected Ca										
Phos (2.4-4.7)										
Mg (1.8-2.5)										
Alb (3.5-4.8)										
PAB (18-38)										
TG (<150)										
AST (15-41)										
ALT (10-40)										
ALP (30-91)										
T bili										
Lipase (22-51)										
NH3 (16-60)										
Intake										
Output										
NGT/ostomy/stool										

TPN Nutrients

IVF: _____
Access: _____

Date										
AA (g)										
Dextrose (g)										
Lipids (g)										
Volume										
Hrs Infused										
Rate										
NaCl (mEq)										
Na Ac (mEq)										
NaPhos (mmol)										
KCl (mEq)										
K Ac (mEq)										
KPhos mmol										
Mg (mEq)										
Ca gluc (mEq)										
MVI (10 ml)										
TE (1 ml)										
Zinc (3 mg)										
Thiamine (100mg)										
Insulin										
Additives & Riders										
GIR (from order)										
Total kcal										
Kcal/Kg										

Electrolyte Guidance:

Corrected Ca = Measured Ca (mg/dL) + [0.8 x (4–serum Alb mg/dL)]

Na	1 – 2 mEq/kg (start 2/kg)	→ needs w/ GI losses
K	10 mEq per 0.1 increase in serum K+	→ needs w/ GI losses, refeeding, meds
Chloride	PRN to maintain acid/base balance	→ needs w/ metabolic alkalosis, volume depletion
Acetate	PRN to maintain acid/base balance	→ needs w/ AKI, metabolic acidosis, bicarb GI losses
Calcium	10 – 15 mEq/day	→ needs w/ high protein intake
Mg	8 – 20 mEq/day	→ needs w/ GI losses, drugs, refeeding
Phos	10 – 40 mmol/day	→ needs w/ high dextrose loads, refeeding

TPN Advancement & Refeeding Syndrome:

- Protein can start at goal. Give half lipids 1st 2 days.
- Choose SMOF if high TG, anticipated prolonged PN, malnourished or critically ill.
- Start dextrose at 100g/d or 50% goal – whichever is less.
- Advance dextrose by 50-100 g/day once lytes stable.
- Add 100 mg thiamine for 1st 7 days or until lytes stable if refeeding risk.
- Continue 100mg/d thiamine for bariatric six patients.
- Renewal lytes:
  - o   If low, increase by 50% of prior day provision; aim for serum K+ level of 4.0
  - o   If trending down but wnl, increase by 25% of prior day provision

GIR = dex g x 1000/1440 min (720 for 12h cycle)/wt kg – should be ≤4-5 mg/kg/min

STORM
NUTRITION
STUDY SUPPORT

https://nutritionstudysupport.com

TPN COMPOSITION GUIDANCE

Electrolyte Guidance:

Volume based on current IVF needs.

Na	1 – 2 mEq/kg *(start 2/kg)*	↑ needs w/ GI losses
K+	1 – 2 mEq/kg *(start conservatively)**	↑ needs w/ GI losses, refeeding, meds
Chloride	PRN to maintain acid/base balance	↑ needs w/ metabolic alkalosis, volume depletion
Acetate	PRN to maintain acid/base balance	↑ needs w/ AKI, metabolic acidosis, bicarb GI losses
Calcium	10 – 15 mEq/day	↑ needs w/ high protein intake
Mg	8 – 20 mEq/day	↑ needs w/ GI losses, drugs, refeeding
Phos	10 – 40 mmol/day	↑ needs w/ high dextrose loads, refeeding

Step-By-Step Guide To Ordering Initial PN Electrolytes:

Volume determination – start with current IVF volume

Start with determining Phos – generally 10-20 mmol initially
- 20 mmol NaPhos = 27 mEq Na (1.33 mEq Na/1 mmol NaPhos)

Sodium can start at 2 mEq/kg or equivalent of ½ NS
- Subtract Na in NaPhos from total Na needs & split Na between NaCl & Na Acetate
- Start at 50/50 split and adjust based on serum Cl & CO_2 levels
- Replace base deficit with acetate; generally, add 10mEq acetate per 1 mm/L CO_2 < 24

Target serum K+ level of 4.0
- 10 mEq of KCl needed to increase serum K^+ by 0.1 mg/dL
- Start K+ conservatively ~ 20-40 mEq – safer to replete with riders

Mg & Calcium can start at low end of above ranges & adjust as needed

Daily Electrolyte Management:

	Too Low	Too High
Sodium	• Increase sodium • Consider increasing fluid	• Increase fluid • Consider decreasing sodium
Chloride	• Increase Cl (preferably as NaCl) & decrease acetate as needed	• Decrease Cl & increase acetate as needed
Acetate	• Replace base deficit with acetate: add 10mEq acetate per 1 mm/L CO_2 < 24	• Decrease or hold acetate
Potassium	• Increase by 10 mEq for every 0.1 increase needed to reach target serum K^* 4.0 • Include any KCl riders in mEq increase need calculation	• Decrease by 10 mEq for every 0.1 decrease needed to reach target serum K^* 4.0 • Hold for K^+ > 5.0
Phosphorus	• Increase NaPhos in PN • If need > 25 mmol, add K^* Phos • If persistently low, check PTH level	• Decrease by 50% or hold • Add enteral phos binders if appropriate
Magnesium	• Each 1g (8 mEq) should ↑ serum Mg by 0.1 mg/dL – equilibrium takes up to 48 hrs	• Decrease by 50% or hold
Calcium	• Add enteral phos binders as able if due to high Phos	• Decrease by 50% or hold

---

TPN Advancement & Refeeding Syndrome:
- Protein can start at goal. Give half lipids 1st 2 days.
- Choose SMOF if high TG, anticipated prolonged PN, malnourished or critically ill.
- Start dextrose at 100g/d or 50% goal – whichever is less.
- Advance dextrose by 33% once lytes stable.
- Add 100 mg thiamine for 1st 7 days or until lytes stable if refeeding risk.
- Continue 100mg/d thiamine for bariatric sx patients.

Order Phos as single salt Na Phos up to 25 mmol.

Any additional Phos needs can be in form of K Phos.

Order K+ as single salt KCl unless additional acetate or Phos needed.

Renewal lytes:
If low, increase by 50% of prior day provision

If trending down but wnl, increase by 25% of prior day provision

Parenteral Nutrition Prescriber Checklist

Patient Name: _____ **MRN:** _____ **Date:** _____

Before Writing the Order

- ☐ Confirmed PN indication; EN/oral options inadequate or not feasible
- ☐ Checked PN appropriateness for current clinical status
- ☐ Verified allergies and adverse reactions to ensure no PN component contraindications

- ☐ Verified access site: ☐ Central line ☐ Peripheral line
- ☐ Line compatibility confirmed; no contraindications noted
- ☐ Confirmed appropriate osmolarity for planned route: _____ mOsm/L

- ☐ Reviewed patient weight: _____ kg | Dosing weight: _____ kg
- ☐ Screened for refeeding risk
- ☐ Labs reviewed and repleted as appropriate
- ☐ TGs checked and < 400 mg/dL prior to initiation of PN lipids
- ☐ Reconciled with other IV fluids—no duplicate electrolytes or fluid overload
- ☐ Reviewed current fluid restrictions and other IV infusions
- ☐ Noted recent propofol, cleviprex, dextrose, or other caloric sources

---

Order Entry & Verification

PN Type: ☐ 2-in-1 (separate lipid) ☐ 3-in-1 (TNA)
Schedule: ☐ Continuous ☐ Cyclic (_____ hrs/day)
Total volume: _____ mL/day | Infusion rate: _____ mL/hr

Macronutrients:
Dextrose: _____ g/day **Amino acids:** _____ g/day **Lipid emulsion:** _____ g/day
- ☐ Final concentration meets stability guidelines: >10% dextrose, > 4% AA, > 2-2.5% lipid
- ☐ Continuous glucose infusion rate does not exceed 5 mg/kg/min (4 mg/kg/min critical care)
- ☐ Cycled glucose infusion rate does not exceed 7 mg/kg/min at peak infusion

Electrolytes:
- ☐ Electrolytes are ordered as complete salts and includes dose
- ☐ Calcium/Phos solubility curve reviewed and within range for stability

Vitamins, Trace Elements, & Additives:
- ☐ Confirmed daily multivitamin and trace element inclusion
- ☐ Thiamine added if RFS risk present (suggest 100 mg daily)
- ☐ Insulin (if ordered) is appropriate
- ☐ Any medications added are confirmed to meet safety and compatibility requirements

Order must be verified by pharmacy as 2nd check prior to compounding

---

Administration & Monitoring

- ☐ Blood glucose monitoring ordered at least Q6H
- ☐ Appropriate lab monitoring ordered for PN management
- ☐ D10W ordered in case PN abruptly discontinued
- ☐ Cycled PN orders include a 1-2 hour taper on start and completion

---

Parenteral Nutrition Order Writing Competency

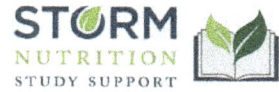

STORM NUTRITION STUDY SUPPORT

RD Name (print): _____

Directions: Evaluator must have advanced knowledge in managing Parenteral Nutrition. Suggest 10 cases reviewed for new RD with < 2 years of experience required for independence in PN order writing.

Patient MRN & Initials:			
Date of Initial Assessment & Follow-up Assessment/Management Duration:			
Competency	**Met**	**Needs Review**	**Comments**
Thorough assessment complete including: client history, anthropometrics, biochemical data, imaging, procedural history, and NFPE.			
Appropriately determined indication for PN			
Appropriately determined appropriate administration route			
Accurately determined dosing weight			
Identify pertinent allergies			
PN ordered correctly via EHR system			
Accurately documented PN infusion rate and total intravenous fluid volume requirement			
Based on completed nutrition assessment accurately determined and ordered macronutrient components of PN			
Identified and accurately ordered vitamins, trace elements, electrolytes, and any other needed additives for PN formulation			
Evaluated for malnutrition and refeeding risk as appropriate			
Demonstrated familiarity with glucose management			
Included any related orders for routine care and monitoring as appropriate			
Complete appropriate PN documentation in patient medical record			
Demonstrated appropriate coordination of care			
Able to appropriately make changes to PN order based on patient's changing clinical condition and tolerance to PN			
Monitored for complications and implemented or recommended appropriate treatment strategies as needed			
Demonstrated appropriate transition between feeding modalities when indicated			
Managed PN product shortages appropriately			

Provider Signature: _____ Date: _____

Evaluator Signature: _____ Date: _____

ABOUT THE AUTHOR

Bridget Storm is a dynamic leader with experience managing both inpatient acute care and outpatient clinical nutrition programs. Bridget volunteers a subject matter expert for the CDR with expertise in nutrition support, critical care and NICU. An advocate for RDN practice at the highest level of licensed scope, Bridget serves on the Delaware State Board of Dietetics and Nutrition. She is an engaged member of AND and ASPEN, where she contributes to the Clinical Practice Guidelines Relief Panel and the Malnutrition Committee. Bridget has presented for FNCE, the AND Center for Lifelong Learning, and multiple AND affiliates on nutrition support, refeeding syndrome, sarcopenic obesity, and Telenutrition. Bridget is a leader on CNSC exam preparation and has self-published a CNSC Study Guide, Nutrition Support Case Studies, and training manuals for nutrition support in NICU, critical care, and GI compromise. Bridget enjoys mentoring providers and teaching nutrition support orientation classes for local internship programs as a means to give back and advance the future of the clinical nutrition.

STORM NUTRITION STUDY SUPPORT

At STORM NUTRITION STUDY SUPPORT, our mission is to empower dietitians for advanced practice career success through comprehensive education, innovative resources, and unwavering support. We are committed to fostering a community where dietitians can enhance their knowledge, skills, and confidence in the dynamic field of nutrition. By providing cutting-edge tools, expert guidance, and collaborative opportunities, we strive to equip dietitians with the capabilities to excel in their professional endeavors, contribute to evidence-based practice, and positively impact individuals' health outcomes. Our dedication to excellence and continuous learning drives us to be the premier partner for dietitians seeking to advance their careers and make a lasting difference in the field of nutrition.

Visit us at https://nutritionstudysupport.com

Social Media Handles:

https://www.instagram.com/storm.nutritionstudysupport

https://www.facebook.com/stormnss

https://www.linkedin.com/in/bridget-storm-ma-rd-ldn-cnsc-b4bb2a19/

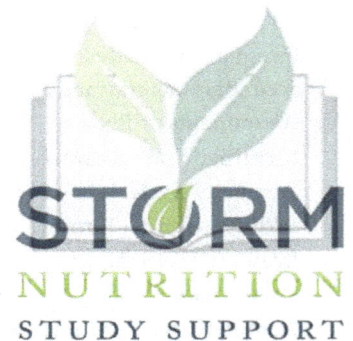

ACKNOWLEDGEMENTS

As the author of this training guide, I want to express my heartfelt thanks to you for taking the time to engage with my work. Your interest in learning and dedication to your advancing your nutrition support skills are truly appreciated. Writing this guide has been a rewarding experience and knowing that it might assist you on your career journey brings me great satisfaction. Thank you for your support and for considering this guide as a resource.

I would like to thank Janice Baker, my most engaged client, for reinforcing the value of the study materials I have created and for motivating me to continue diversifying my product portfolio.

I would like to thank Linda Doyle, my colleague and good friend, for all of her support on both a professional and personal level. Your recognition of the work I am trying to accomplish gives me the encouragement to continue creating educational resources.

Finally, I would like to extend my deepest thanks to my husband, David Storm, for his patience with my long hours and his support of "The Side Hustle".

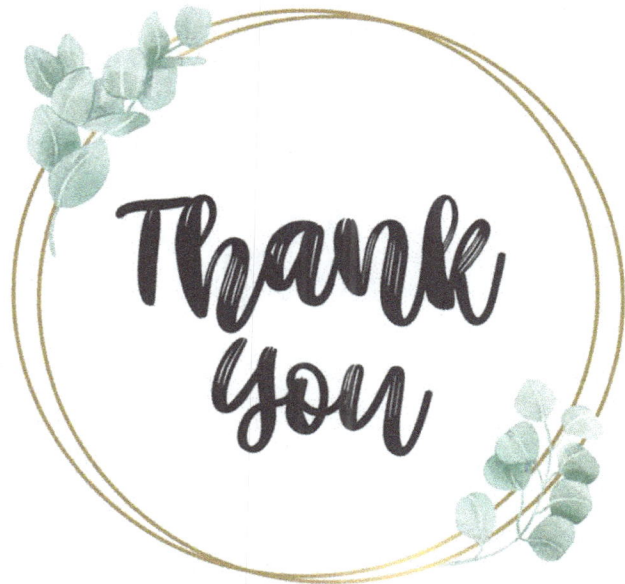

www.ingramcontent.com/pod-product-compliance
Lightning Source LLC
Chambersburg PA
CBHW081110220326
41598CB00038B/7306